Acronyms & Synonyms in Medical Imaging

Professor David Allison BSc MD MRCP FRCR

Director and Professor of Diagnostic Radiology,
Department of Diagnostic Radiology, The Royal Postgraduate Medical School,
Hammersmith, London

Dr Nicola Strickland BM BCh MA Hons(Oxon)
MRCP(UK) FRCR
Senior Lecturer and Consultant Radiologist, Department of
Diagnostic Radiology, The Royal Postgraduate Medical School
Hammersmith Hospital, London

I S I S
MEDICAL
M E D I A

Oxford

© 1996 by Isis Medical Media Ltd.
58 St Aldates
Oxford OX1 1ST, UK

First published 1996

British Library Cataloguing in Publication Data. A catalogue record for this title is available from the British Library

ISBN 1 899066 10 1

Allison D. (David)
Acronyms & Synonyms in Medical Imaging
David Allison and Nicola Strickland

Always refer to the manufacturer's Prescribing Information before prescribing drugs cited in this book.

Typeset by
Advance Typesetting Ltd, Oxon, UK

Printed and bound by
Redwood Books, Wilts, UK

Distributed by
Times Mirror International Publishers
Customer Service Centre, Unit 1, 3 Sheldon Way, Larkfield, Aylesford, Kent ME20 6SF, UK

Preface

The idea of writing this book evolved from the editors' involvement with the installation of a PACS (picture archive and communication system, q.v.) at Hammersmith Hospital. This introduced us as medics to a bewildering gamut of acronyms concerning the technological aspects of medical imaging. We began compiling our own glossary of these terms for personal use, and then realised just how many acronyms, synonyms and abbreviations are in daily use throughout clinical practice, particularly on X-ray and other request forms. We have attempted to collect and cross-reference as many of these as possible to compile a dictionary which we hope will benefit not only doctors, radiographers, nurses, physiotherapists, medical secretaries, receptionists and ward clerks, but also those many other groups who regularly use medical terms such as hospital managers, physicists, medical suppliers and medical publishers.

Within the constraints imposed by the need for brevity and accuracy we have endeavoured to make the explanation of terms as simple and straightforward as possible.

Despite our best efforts there will undoubtedly be many omissions from this work and new acronyms are being coined all the time. We would greatly welcome any contributions from readers concerning acronyms, synonyms or abbreviations in their own specialist fields that we have not mentioned, so that we can make the next edition of this work more comprehensive and ultimately expand it into a more general work embracing the entire discipline of medicine.

David Allison
Nicola Strickland

List of Contributors

Dr med. Thomas Albrecht
Dr Stuart Coley, MB ChB MRCP(UK)
Dr Catherine Ramsey, BSc MB BS MRCP(UK)
Dr Ruth Williamson, BSc MB BS MRCP(UK)

Department of Radiology, Royal Postgraduate Medical School, Hammersmith Hospital, London W12 0NN, UK

and

Dr Thomas Lee Pope, Jr, MD (North American advisor)

Professor of Radiology and Orthopedics, Bowman Gray School of Medicine, 2nd Floor Meads Hall, Medical Center Boulevard, Winston-Salem, NC 27157-1088, USA

How to use this book

Wherever possible each entry in this book is broken down into five levels:-

1. Common abbreviation or Acronym   **PACS**
    (US equivalent shown in brackets)

2. Full text entry   **Picture archiving and communications
                                          system**

3. Full definition   A hospital-wide network for generating,
                                          viewing, archiving and retrieving digital
                                          images and their associated reports.

4. Synonym   IMACS

5. Cross reference   (*see HIS, MDIS, RIS*)

A

α-1 Antitryp
Alpha 1 antitrypsin
Enzyme (protease inhibitor) synthesized by the liver. Deficiency is associated with liver disease and lower lobe emphysema.

α-1 AT
Alpha 1 antitrypsin
See under α-1 Antitryp.

α decay
Alpha decay
Form of radioactive decay which occurs in heavy nuclei. It results in the emission of an alpha particle (α particle).
α emission

α emission
Alpha emission
See under α decay.

αfp
Alphafetoprotein
A protein produced by the embryonic yolk sac and fetal liver; measured during screening for fetal abnormalities and some adult tumours.
αFP, afp, aFP

αFP
Alphafetoprotein
See under αfp.
afp, aFP

α-IFN
Alpha interferon
Lymphokines (glycoproteins) released by B lymphocytes in response to viral infections. Used in treatment of malignancy, especially hairy cell leukaemia.
(see IFN)

α-MSH
Alpha melanocyte stimulating hormone
Peptide produced from the precursor adrenocorticotrophic hormone (ACTH) in melanotrophs of the pituitary pars intermedia.
(see β–MSH, γ–MSH)

α motor nerve/neurone
Alpha motor nerve/neurone
Motor nerve/neurone directly innervating muscle.
LMN

α particle
Alpha particle
Helium nucleus consisting of two protons and two neutrons which is emitted during alpha decay (α decay).

α radiation
Alpha radiation
Stream of alpha particles (α particles).
α ray

α ray
Alpha ray
See under α radiation.

a
Area
Two dimensional measurement of space.

A
Ampere
SI unit of electric current (I).

A
Atrial branch
Branch of the right coronary artery.

A
Mass number
Total number of protons and neutrons within the nucleus of an atom.
(see Z)

A₂
Aortic valve
Component of second heart sound.

AA
Abdominal aorta
Abdominal part of the main artery of the body.
(see Ao, AO)

AA
Alcoholics Anonymous
Voluntary organization for the rehabilitation of alcoholics.

AA
Amyloid A
Extracellular deposition of the fibrous protein amyloid A, secondary to coexisting (commonly chronic) disease.
(see AL)

AA
Aortic arch
Part of the thoracic aorta which connects the ascending and descending aorta.
(see Ao, AO)

AA
Atlantoaxial
Pertaining to the two upper cervical vertebrae: atlas and axis.

AA
Autoantibodies / autoantibody
Antibodies formed in response to subject's own protein(s).
(see Ab)

AAA
Abdominal aortic aneurysm
Abnormal dilatation of the intra-abdominal aorta.
(see AA)

AAA
Acute anxiety attack
Sudden onset 'panic attack'.

AAC
Antibiotic-associated (pseudomembranous) colitis
Diarrhoeal illness which occurs following treatment with broad-spectrum antibiotics; associated with strains of *Clostridium difficile*.
AAPC, PMC

AAL
Anterior axillary line
Imaginary anatomical line extending vertically downwards from the anterior axillary fold.

AAo
Ascending aorta
Segment of the thoracic aorta which extends from the left ventricular outlet to the aortic arch.
(see AA, Ao)

AAPC
Antibiotic-associated pseudomembranous colitis
See under AAC.
PMC

Ab
Antibiotic
Antimicrobial agent that kills or damages bacteria.
ATB

Ab
Antibody
Protein essential to immune defence.
(see AA)

AB
Abnormal beliefs
Feature of psychotic illness.

AB
Apex beat
Most inferior and lateral point at which the cardiac impulse is palpable.

AB
Asbestos body
Asbestos particle, identified histologically which indicates previous exposure to potentially hazardous asbestos fibres.

ABA
Allergic bronchopulmonary aspergillosis
Hypersensitivity to *Aspergillus fumigatus*; demonstrated by asthma-like symptoms, positive precipitins and typical chest radiographic features.
ABPA

ABA
Antibacterial activity
Properties of a preparation that halts the growth of, or destroys, bacteria.

ABC
Acalculous biliary colic
Upper abdominal discomfort caused by painful contraction of the biliary tree in the absence of gallstones.
(see GB,GS)

ABC
Airway, breathing, circulation
List of priorities in cardiopulmonary resuscitation (CPR).
(see AR, BLS, ECM)

ABC
Aneurysmal bone cyst
Expansile lesion of bone containing blood-filled cystic cavities.

abd
Abduction
Movement of a body-part away from the midline.

ABE
Acute bacterial endocarditis
Acute infection of the endothelium lining the heart, commonly in relation to an abnormal or prosthetic heart valve.
(see BE, IE, SBE)

ABG

Arterial blood gases
Biochemical analysis of arterial blood, including oxygen and carbon dioxide levels, and acid–base status.

ABMT

Autologous bone marrow transplantation
Bone marrow replacement from another person.

Abn.

Abnormal

ABO.

Abortion
Termination of a pregnancy.
Abor

ABO

ABO system
The major classification of blood groups. (A,B,O and AB).

Abor.

Abortion
See under ABO.

ABP

Arterial blood pressure
Arterial pressure of blood, usually measured with a sphygmomanometer during both the systolic and diastolic phases of the cardiac cycle.
BP
(see HT)

ABPA

Allergic bronchopulmonary aspergillosis
See under ABA.

ABPC

Antibody-producing cell
Immunocompetent cell (lymphocyte) capable of antibody synthesis.

ABPI

Association of British Pharmaceuticals in Industry
A body which represents British drug manufacturing. It compiles the data sheet compendium of pharmaceuticals.

ABR

Absolute bed rest
Patient strictly confined to bed.
SCR

ABT

Autologous blood transfusion
Intravenous (IV) administration of a patient's own blood to him/herself to treat anaemia/ blood loss after an operation/procedure.
(see BTx)

ABU

Asymptomatic bacteriuria
Bacteria detected in the urine without associated symptoms. Relevant to obstetric practice.
(see AUA)

ABVD

Adriamycin, bleomycin, vinblastine and dacarbazine
Chemotherapy regimen.

a.c.

Alternating current
Electric current reversing its direction with a constant frequency (f).
AC
(see DC)

a.c.

ante cibum
Before meals (literally before food).
Ant. prand.

A-C

Acromioclavicular
Joint, ligament or capsule between the clavicle and acromion.
AC, ac

AC

Abdominal circumference
Girth measurement, usually of a fetus in utero, measured by ultrasound.

AC

Abdominal compression
Pressure applied to the abdomen; used during intravenous urography to distend the pelvicaliceal systems.

AC

Acute cholecystitis
Acute inflammation of the gallbladder causing fever and abdominal pain.
(see GB)

AC, ac

Acromioclavicular
See under A-C.

AC
Alcoholic cirrhosis
Diffuse hepatocellular necrosis, with subsequent fibrosis and nodule formation following chronic alcohol abuse.

AC
Alternating current
See under a.c.
(see DC, f)

AC
Anticoagulant
Pharmacological agent which inhibits the normal blood clotting mechanisms.
(see ACT)

AC
Ascending colon
Part of the right hemicolon.

ACA
Anticentromere antibody
An antibody found in patients with CREST syndrome.

ACA
Anterior cerebral artery
Branch of the internal carotid artery which supplies the frontal lobes of the brain.
(see ACOM)

ACC
Articular chondrocalcinosis
Cartilaginous calcification of joints, seen in a number of medical conditions.

ACD
Acid citrate dextrose
An anticoagulant used in stored blood.

ACD
Anaemia of chronic disorders
Normochromic, normocytic anaemia found in chronic infections, inflammatory and collagen vascular disorders and malignant disease.

ACD
Allergic contact dermatitis
Inflammatory skin reaction following direct contact with an allergen.

AC–DC
Bisexual (slang)
(see B & D, SM)

ACE
Angiotensin-converting enzyme
Enzyme responsible for production of angiotensin II: a powerful endogenous vasoconstrictor.
5-ACE
(see ACEI)

ACEI
Angiotensin-converting enzyme inhibitor
Drug producing vasodilatation by blocking ACE activity. Used currently in the management of cardiac failure, hypertension, myocardial infarction and diabetic nephropathy.

Ach (ACh)
Acetylcholine
Central and peripheral neurotransmitter.

AchE
Acetylcholinesterase
Enzyme of the synaptic cleft which inactivates acetylcholine (neurotransmitter).

Ach 'esterase
Acetylcholinesterase
See under AchE.

Ach 'esterase I
Acetylcholinesterase inhibitor
Drug acting on the synaptic cleft which prevents acetylcholine (neurotransmitter) inactivation.

Acid phos (ph).
Acid phosphatase
Enzyme present in prostate, liver, red cells, platelets and bone. Elevated serum levels are indicative of prostate carcinoma.
ACP, AP

ACKD
Acquired cystic kidney disease
Renal cysts forming in the native kidneys of patients on long-term dialysis, or with a renal transplant in situ.

ACL
Anterior cruciate ligament
Central knee ligament between femur and tibia which contributes to joint stability.
(see PCL)

ACLS
Advanced cardiac life support
System of emergency management of patients with acute cardiovascular disease.

ACOM
> **Anterior communicating artery**
> Artery connecting the two anterior cerebral
> arteries forming part of the circle of Willis.
> (see ACA)

ACOP
> **Approved code of practice**
> National British legal document accompanying
> the Ionizing Radiation Regulations 1985
> (IRR 1985). Gives details on compliance with
> the regulations.

ACP
> **Acid phosphatase**
> See under Acid phos (ph).
> AP

ACR
> **American College of Radiologists**

ACR-NEMA
> **American College of Radiologists–National**
> **Electric Manufacturers Association**
> Refers to standards for medical digital image
> communication developed jointly by ACR and
> NEMA.

ACT
> **Anticoagulant therapy**
> Treatment inhibiting normal blood clotting.
> (see AC)

ACTH
> **Adrenocorticotrophic hormone**
> Anterior pituitary gland hormone which
> stimulates the adrenal cortex.
> ADCH

A/D
> **Analogue to digital conversion**
> Means of converting an analogue signal into a
> digital one.

AD
> **Alzheimer's dementia**
> Most commonly acquired cerebral
> degenerative disease.
> ASD, DAT

AD
> **Autosomal dominant**
> Genetic situation in which a single harmful
> mutation in one allele will manifest itself as
> disease.

ADC
> **Analogue to digital conversion**
> See under A/D.

ADC
> **AIDS dementia complex**
> Progressive subcortical dementia in an
> acquired immunodeficiency syndrome (AIDS)
> patient.

ADCH
> **Adrenocorticotrophic hormone**
> See under ACTH.

AD converter
> **Analogue to digital converter**
> Electronic component of an imaging system
> which transforms analogue to digital signals.
> (see DA converter)

add.
> **Adduction**
> Movement of a body part towards the midline.

ADEM
> **Acute disseminated encephalomyelitis**
> Immune-mediated, widespread demyelination
> of cerebral white matter following a
> viral infection.

AdenoCa
> **Adenocarcinoma**
> Malignant proliferation of 'glandular' cells.

ADH
> **Anti-diuretic hormone**
> Posterior pituitary hormone which regulates
> water homeostasis.
> AVP
> (see DI)

ADL
> **Activities of daily living**
> Includes washing, dressing, cooking and
> shopping.

ADL
> **Annual dose limit**
> Legally-stated constraints on the ionizing
> radiation dose which is received in
> occupational exposure and by the
> general public.

ADP
> **Adenosine diphosphate**
> Nucleotide produced by hydrolysis of ATP;
> involved in energy metabolism.
> (see ATP)

ADPD

Autosomal dominant polycystic disease
Autosomal-dominant hereditary disease causing renal parenchymal cyst formation and ultimately in renal failure. Associated with pancreatic, splenic and hepatic cysts and intracranial aneurysms. Usually presents in adult life.
ACPC, APD, APKD, PCKD

ADR

Adrenaline (US: epinephrine)
Catecholamine produced by the adrenal medulla.
(*see* DOPA, DOPamine, NADR)

ADR

Adverse drug reaction
An unwanted side effect of a drug.

ADSL

Asymmetrical digital single line
Means of sending digital images. The line allows one way data traffic only.

ADT

Admission, discharge and transfer
An information function which documents patient details on a hospital information system (HIS).

A & E

Accident and emergency
Casualty department.
Cas

AE

Air entry
Lung ventilation, assessed clinically by the auscultation of breath sounds and the observation of chest-wall movements.

AE

Atrial ectopic (beat)
Early contraction of the atrial heart chambers.
APB, APC, APD

AEF

Amyloid-enhancing factor
An extract of amyloidotic tissue injected intravenously (IV) into mice to render them susceptible to AA amyloid as an experimental disease model.

AF

Amniotic fluid
Fluid surrounding the fetus, contained by the amniotic membranes.
(*see* AFV)

AF

Atrial fibrillation
Common cardiac arrhythmia, characterized by disorganized atrial activity with an irregular ventricular response.

AFB

Acid fast bacilli
Causative bacterium in tuberculosis (consumption).

AFLP

Acute fatty liver of pregnancy
Fatty infiltration of the liver during pregnancy. May present with hepatic failure.

AFM

After fatty meal
Term used during an ultrasonic or cholecystographic examination of the gall bladder which normally contracts after fatty food has been eaten.
(*see* CSG)

afp

Alphafetoprotein
See under αfp.
αFP, aFP, AFP

aFP

Alphafetoprotein
See under αfp.
αFP, afp, AFP

AFP

Adiabatic fast passage
Technique in magnetic resonance imaging for producing a rotation of the magnetic vector by varying the frequency of an irradiating radio wave.

AFP

Alphafetoprotein
See under αfp.
αFP, afp, aFP

AFV

Amniotic fluid volume
Amount of liquor surrounding the developing fetus. Its ultrasonic assessment forms part of the biophysical profile score (BPS).
(*see* AF)

Ag

Antigen
Molecular structure against which an antibody can be raised.

Ag
Silver
Metal used in radiographic film, causes blackening.

Ag–Ab
Antigen–antibody
Complex of antigen and its corresponding antibody.

AgBr
Silver bromide
Main component of radiographic film emulsion.

AGC
Automatic gain control
Function of an ultrasound machine which removes the operator-dependent time gain compensation control, to make the images more reproducible.
TGC

AGN
Acute glomerulonephritis
Type of glomerulonephritis (GN) characterized by the rapid onset of a nephritic syndrome (typically after streptococcal infection).
(*see PSGN*)

AHCD
Acquired hepatocellular degeneration
Irreversible neurodegenerative syndrome that occurs with many types of chronic liver disease.

AI
Aortic incompetence
'Leaky' aortic valve.
AR

AI
Artificial insemination
Instrumental introduction of semen into the vagina.
(*see AID, AIH*)

AI
Artificial intelligence
Computer-based technology that can simulate characteristics of human intelligence. Such computer programs are capable of learning from experience in order to solve problems.

AICA
Anterior inferior cerebellar artery
First branch of the basilar artery supplying the cerebellum.

AID
Artificial insemination by a donor
Artificial insemination using semen from a donor other than the recipient's husband.
(*see AI, AIH*)

AIDP
Acute inflammatory demyelinating polyneuritis
Otherwise known as Guillain–Barré syndrome (GBS). Characterized by subacute ascending paralysis with areflexia but only mild sensory deficit. There is a marked elevation of the cerebrospinal fluid protein level.

AIDS
Acquired immunodeficiency syndrome
Syndrome of opportunistic disease in immunocompromised seropositive human immunodeficiency virus (HIV) individuals.
(*see AZT*)

AIH
Artificial insemination by the husband.
Artificial insemination using semen donated by the husband of the recipient.
(*see AI, AID*)

AIHA
Autoimmune haemolytic anaemia
Condition of diverse aetiology characterized by anaemia caused by an immune-mediated destruction of red blood cells.

AIIS
Anterior inferior iliac spine
Bony prominence on the lower part of the front of the iliac bone.
(*see ASIS*)

AIN
Acute interstitial nephritides
Group of acute renal diseases, characterized by an immunologically-based glomerulonephritis (GN).

AION
Anterior ischaemic optic neuropathy
Sudden onset unilateral painless visual loss due to infarction of the short posterior ciliary arteries supplying the optic disc. May be of atherosclerotic or of vasculitic aetiology.

AIP

Acute intermittent porphyria
Uroporphyrin I synthetase deficiency causing drug-induced visceral pain, paralysis, behavioural disturbance and autonomic dysfunction.
IAP
(see ALA, PBG)

AIUM

American Institute of Ultrasound in Medicine
Professional organization of ultrasonographers and sonologists; publishes *Journal of Ultrasound in Medicine*.

AJ

Ankle jerk
Involuntary contraction of gastrocnemius muscles in response to sudden passive stretching of the Achilles tendon.

AJR

American Journal of Roentgenology
Monthly peer-reviewed journal of the American College of Radiologists (ACR).
Am. J. Roentgenol.

AKA

Above knee amputation
(see BKA)

AKA

Also known as
(see OKA)

AL

Amyloid L
Extracellular deposition of the protein amyloid L, in the absence of coexisting disease.
(see AA)

Al

Aluminium
Metal commonly used for X-ray filtration. Also used in xeroradiography plates.
(see Al$_2$O$_3$, Se)

ALA

5-Aminolaevulinate
Precursor in the haem synthesis pathway. Acts as a urinary marker for acute intermittent porphyria (AIP).

ALARA

As low as is reasonably achievable
Fundamental principle of radiation protection whereby the dose of ionizing radiation is kept to a minimum during any procedure.

ALD

Adrenoleukodystrophy
Inherited error of a single peroxisomal enzyme, characterized by cerebral white matter demyelination and endocrine dysfunction.

ALD

Alcoholic liver disease
Spectrum of diseases affecting the liver caused by excessive alcohol intake.

ALF

Acute liver failure
Acute hepatic dysfunction, of diverse aetiology.

ALI

Annual limit on intake
Limit of yearly intake, ingested or inhaled, of a particular radioisotope by hospital staff, as stated by the Ionizing Radiation Regulations 1985 (IRR 1985).

Alk. Phos.

Alkaline phosphatase
Enzyme present in liver, bone and placenta. A raised serum level indicates either liver or bone disease, or pregnancy.
ALP, SALP

ALL

Acute lymphocytic leukaemia (acute lymphoblastic leukaemia)
Neoplastic proliferation of bone marrow lymphoid precursor cells.

Allo-BMT

Allogeneic bone marrow transplantation
Bone marrow engraftment between genetically non-identical individuals.
(see auto-BMT)

Al$_2$O$_3$

Aluminium oxide
Insulating layer in a xeroradiography plate.
(see Al, Se)

ALP

Alkaline phosphatase
See under Alk. Phos.
SALP

ALP

Anterior lobe of pituitary
One of the two lobes of the brain's pituitary gland.
Ant. pit., AP
(see PLP)

ALS

Amyotrophic lateral sclerosis
Neurological disease characterized by progressive muscle weakness, limb and truncal atrophy, and bulbar symptoms and signs.
MND

ALT

Alanine aminotransferase
Hepatocellular enzyme. Elevated serum levels indicate liver disease.
SGPT

ALVF

Acute left ventricular failure
Inability of the heart's left ventricle to pump blood adequately. Results in pulmonary congestion and/or low systemic output.
(see HF)

AM

Acute marginal artery
Branch of the right coronary artery.

AM

Adnexal mass
Tumour situated around the ovaries or Fallopian tubes.

AMA

Antimitochondrial antibody
Antibody used as a marker for autoimmune disease of the liver especially primary biliary cirrhosis (PBC).

AMC

Arthrogryphosis multiplex congenita
Heterogeneous group of disorders characterized by multiple joint contractures Amyoplasia congenita.

AMI

Anterior myocardial infarction
Ischaemic death of cardiac tissue resulting from left anterior coronary arterial occlusion.
(see TAMI)

Am. J. Roentgenol.

American Journal of Roentgenology
See under AJR.

AML

Acute myeloid leukaemia
Neoplastic proliferation of bone marrow granulocyte precursor cells.

AML

Angiomyolipoma
Benign mesenchymal tumour of the kidney, multiple in tuberose (tuberous) sclerosis.

AML

Anterior mitral leaflet
One of the two leaflets of the heart's mitral valve.
aMVL

A-Mode

Amplitude mode
Linear ultrasound technique recording static information relating to the depth of a reflecting object and the magnitude of its reflected signal.

AMP

Adenosine monophosphate
Nucleotide involved in cellular energy metabolism and nucleotide synthesis.

AMS

α amylase
Enzyme produced by pancreas and salivary glands. Elevated serum levels are indicative of acute pancreatitis.

AMS

Amyotrophic lateral sclerosis
Nervous system disease characterized by a progressive loss of upper and lower motor neurones. Causes muscle wasting, weakness, spastic paresis and eventually respiratory failure.

aMVL

Anterior mitral valve leaflet
See under AML.

A/N

Antenatal
During pregnancy.
AN

AN

Antenatal
See under A/N.

AN

Acoustic neuroma
Tumour of the vestibulocochlear nerve (eighth cranial nerve).

AN

Anorexia nervosa
Eating disorder, especially of young women, who starve themselves owing to a disordered perception of body image.

AN
Autonomic neuropathy
Dysfunction of the body's 'involuntary' nervous system.

AN
Avascular necrosis
Ischaemic bone cell death.
AVN

A.N. Other
Another
Putative initial and surname of an unknown or anonymous person.
(see JD)

ANA
Anti-nuclear antibody
An antibody found in some diseases of probable autoimmune aetiology, e.g. systemic sclerosis (SS), systemic lupus erythematosus (SLE), Sjörgen's syndrome.

ANC
Absolute neutrophil count
Quantitation of the circulating white neutrophil cell population.

ANCA
Anti-neutrophil cytoplasmic antibody
Immunological marker for vasculitic diseases.
(see c-ANCA, p-ANCA)

Angio.
Angiographic suite
Department in which angiographic studies are conducted.

Angio.
Angiography
Technique for imaging blood vessels.

Ank. Spond.
Ankylosing spondylitis
Inflammatory spondyloarthritis of the spine and sacro-iliac joints, which occurs in HLA B27 individuals, mainly males.
AS

ANOVA
Analysis of variance
Statistical test comparing the means of three or more groups.

ant., ANT.
Anterior
Used in anatomical descriptions to denote ventral situation; in front; in front of.
(see inf., post., sup.)

Ant. pit.
Anterior pituitary
See under ALP.
AP
(see post. pit.)

Ant. prand.
Ante prandium
Before meals.
ac

Ant. tib.
Anterior tibial
Anatomical term for compartment, vessels or nerve of the front of the lower leg.

anti-CEA
Anti-carcinoembryonic antigen antibody
Monoclonal antibody which can be labelled with Indium -111 and used to image tumours in nuclear medicine.
(see ^{111}In)

Anti-D
Anti-D immunoglobulin
Immunoglobulin administered to Rhesus-negative mothers to prevent them from forming antibodies to fetal Rhesus-positive cells which enter the maternal circulation following childbirth or abortion.

Anti-GBM
Anti-glomerular basement membrane
Autoantibody directed against the renal membrane between the vascular endothelium and glomerulus. Causes renal disease and may be associated with pulmonary haemorrhage (Goodpasture's disease).
(see GBM)

Anti-RNP
Anti-ribonucleoprotein antibody
Antibody to a nuclear ribonucleoprotein antigen; high circulating titres characterize mixed connective tissue diseases (MCTD).
(see RNP)

A/O
Alert and orientated
Indicates patient had no clouding of consciousness at time of examination.

AO (US: AAO, AA$_0$)
Ascending aorta
Segment of the thoracic aorta extending from the left ventricular outlet to the aortic arch.
(see AA, Ao, Asc)

Ao
Aorta
Main artery of the body.
(see AA, AO, C of A)

AOB
Alcohol on breath
Alcohol smelt on a patient's breath indicating recent ingestion.
(see C$_2$H$_5$OH, DTs, EtOH, FAS)

AOD
Adult onset diabetes
Diabetes mellitus, usually type 2 or non-insulin dependent diabetes, the onset of which occurs in adulthood.
AODM

AOD
Arterial occlusive disease
Blockage of the arterial vascular tree, either acutely or chronically, by embolus or thrombus (blood clot). Commonly due to atheroma but also occurs in inflammatory conditions and other disorders.
(see AS, ASCVD, ASHD, ASPVD, PVD)

AODM
Adult onset diabetes mellitus
See under AOD.

AOE
Admission order entry
Software application allowing input of patient demographic data and exam schedules into a computerized system, such as a PACS (picture archive and communications system), HIS (hospital information system) or RIS (radiological information system) from a remote site.

AOM
Acute otitis media
Acute, painful, infective inflammation of the middle ear cavity.
(see COM, CSOM, OE)

AOT
Andersson Olsson table
Automatic cut film changer previously used for angiography. Manufactured by Siemens Ltd.

AOT
'Head over heels'
Euphemistic description of the nature of a patient's fall.

AoV
Aortic valve
Cardiac valve which normally ensures unidirectional blood flow from the left ventricle into the ascending aorta.

A/P
Antepartum
Prior to childbirth.
AP

AP
Acid phosphatase
See under Acid phosph.
ACP

AP
Acute pancreatitis
Acute episode of pancreatic inflammation, commonly presenting as abdominal pain. Alcohol and biliary calculi are common precipitating causes.

AP
Angina pectoris
Chest pain caused by coronary arterial ischaemia.

AP
Antepartum
See under A/P.

AP
Anterior pituitary
See under ALP.
Ant. pit.

AP
Antero posterior
From front to back; defines the direction in which the X-ray beam traverses the body.
(see PA)

APB
Atrial premature beat(s)
See under AE.
APC, APD

APC
Antigen presenting cell
Immunocompetent white cell integral to the immune response.

APC
Atrial premature contraction
See under AE.
APB, APD

APCD

Adult polycystic disease
See under APDP.
APD, APKD, PCKD

APD

Aminohydroxypropylidenediphosphonate (disodium pamidronate)
Drug used in the treatment of hypercalcaemia, especially in malignancy.

APD

Atrial premature depolarization
Early electrical stimulation and contraction of the atrial chambers of the heart.
AE, APB, APC

APD

Automated peritoneal dialysis
A variant of continuous ambulatory peritoneal dialysis (CAPD) renal replacement therapy performed at night during sleep. Automatic cycler equipment dispenses and drains the dialysis fluid.
(*see CCPD, IPD*)

APER

Abdomino–perineal excision of rectum
Surgical procedure for the treatment of low rectal carcinomas (below the level of the peritoneal reflection).
APR

APG

Antegrade pyelogram
Radiographic study of the renal collecting system in which contrast medium is injected directly into the renal pelvis.

APH

***Ante partum* haemorrhage**
Bleeding *per vaginam* after 28 weeks gestation.

API

Applications programming interface
Software designed to make a computer's facilities accessible to an application program.

APKD

Adult polycystic disease
See under ADPD.
APCD, APD, PCKD

APN

Acute pyelonephritis
Acute infection of renal parenchyma and collecting system.

Apo. A

Apoprotein A
Protein carried by chylomicrons and high-density lipoprotein (HDL). It is necessary as a cofactor for lecithin–cholesterol acyltransferase (LCAT).

APORF

Acute postoperative renal failure
Renal dysfunction following surgery.

APR

Abdomino–perineal resection
See under APER.

APR

Acute phase reaction
Increase in serum proteins associated with active infection/inflammation.
(*see CRP*)

APS

Antiphospholipid syndrome
A type of systemic lupus erythematosus (SLE) where circulating antiphospholipid (anticardiolipin) autoantibodies are present (previously known as lupus anticoagulant from their action *in vitro*). *In vivo* they predispose to thrombosis and associated phenomena including recurrent abortions.

APSAC

Anisoylated plasminogen–streptokinase activator complex
Thrombolytic agent anistreplase.

APSGN

Acute post-streptococcal glomerulonephritis
Acute glomerulonephritis (AG) secondary to pharyngeal or cutaneous infection with group A β-haemolytic *streptococci*.
PSGN

APTT

Activated partial thromboplastin time
Measurement of a component of the blood coagulation mechanism.

APUD

Amine precursor uptake and decarboxylation
Descriptive term for cells which manufacture polypeptides and biogenic amines serving as hormones or neurotransmitters.

APSCVIR

Asian Pacific Society of Cardiovascular and Interventional Radiology
(*see BSIR, CIRSE, JSAIR, SCVIR, WAIS*)

APVR

Anomalous pulmonary venous return
Developmental failure of the connection
between the pulmonary veins, and the right
atrium.
(*see HAPVD, PAPVD, TAPVD*)

APW

Aortopulmonary window
Anatomical space between aortic arch above
and main pulmonary artery below. Site of
pathological mediastinal lymph nodes.

AR

Allergic rhinitis
Over-production of nasal secretions in response
to an allergic stimulus (e.g. pollen).

AR

Aortic regurgitation
See under AI.

AR

Artificial respiration/assisted respiration
The maintenance of breathing by external
means when natural breathing has ceased or
is insufficient to maintain adequate gas
exchange.
(*see ABC, BLS, CPR, ECM, IMV, IPPV*)

AR

Autosomal recessive
Genetic disorder in which two abnormal genes
are required for the condition to be manifest.

ARA

Anal-rectal agenesis / anorectal agenesis
Failure of development of the anus and
rectum.

ARC

AIDS-related complex
Prodromal phase of acquired immunodeficiency
syndrome (AIDS) with generalized
lymphadenopathy.
LAS

ARC

Archive controller
System controlling the organization and
function of a long term storage repository of
digital images.

ARDMS

**American Registry of Diagnostic Medical
Sonographers**
Professional body administering certification
examination in ultrasonography.

ARDS

Adult respiratory distress syndrome
Acute respiratory insufficiency of diverse
aetiology. Characterized by refractory
hypoxaemia owing to non-cardiac pulmonary
oedema.
(*see RDS*)

ARF

Acute renal failure
A rapid deterioration in kidney function
(occurring in days or weeks), resulting in the
inadequate elimination of toxic metabolic
products.
RPRF
(*see ATN, CRF, RF*)

ARM

Artificial rupture of membranes
Medical intervention to induce labour by
rupturing the amniotic membranes with a
small hook (amnihook) introduced through
the cervix.
AROM
(*see IOL, ROM, SROM*)

AROM

Artificial rupture of membranes
See under ARM.

ARPD

Autosomal recessive polycystic disease
A disorder with autosomal recessive
inheritance characterized by small cysts and
fibrous tissue in the kidneys and liver.
IPCD

ARR

Automatic repeat request
A technique used for error control over a
transmission line.

ARSAC

**Administration of Radioactive Substances
Advisory Committee**
UK committee responsible for advising health
ministers on the granting of certificates for the
administration of radioactive substances.

ARSAC regulations

**Administration of Radioactive Substances
Advisory Committee regulations**
National British legislation on radiation
protection in nuclear medicine; The
Medicines Regulations 1978.

AS

Ankylosing spondylitis
See under Ank. Spond.

AS
Aortic stenosis
Narrowing of the cardiac aortic valve resulting in obstructed left ventricular outflow.
AVS

AS
Arteriosclerosis/otic
Condition in which plaques of abnormal fat, cells and debris, often with calcification, are deposited in the heart and peripheral vascular tree causing progressive vascular occlusion.
(see AOD, ASCVD, ASHD, ASPVD, PVD)

5-ASA
5-Aminosalicyclic acid / mesalazine
Drug used for the treatment of ulcerative colitis.

ASAP
As soon as possible
(see PDQ)

ASC
Asthma symptom checklist
Aid to asthma management, used for assessing the severity of the disease.

asc.
Ascending
(see AO)

ASCII
American standard code for information interchange
An internationally accepted code convention where each character in the Western alphabet, numerals and typewriter keyboard characters have a unique 7-bit pattern.

ASCVD
Arteriosclerotic cardiovascular disease
See under AS.
(see AOD, ASHD, ASPVD, PVD)

ASD
Alzheimer's senile dementia
See under AD.
DAT

ASD
Arthritis syphilitica deformans
Destructive, deforming joint disease associated with tertiary syphilis ($3^0\Sigma$).

ASD
Atrial septal defect
Absence or partial deficiency of the wall between the right and left atrial chambers of the heart.
(see CHD, VSD)

ASDH
Acute sub-dural haemorrhage
Bleeding into the sub-dural space of the meninges presenting acutely.

ASFAIK
As far as I know

ASH
Asymmetrical septal hypertrophy
Presentation of hypertrophic obstructive cardiomyopathy (HOCM).
IHSS

ASHD
Arteriosclerotic heart disease
See under AS.
(see AOD, ASCVD, ASHD, ASPVD, PVD)

ASIC
Application specific integrated circuit
A circuit custom-designed to carry out a specific function.

ASIS
Anterior superior iliac spine
Bony prominence on upper part of the front of the iliac bone.
(see AIIS)

ASO
Anti-streptolysin O
Serum antibody against streptolysin-O.
(see ASOT)

ASOT
Anti-streptolysin O titre
Measurement of serum antibodies to infer past or present infection with Streptococcus e.g. rheumatic fever.
(see ASO)

ASPVD
Arteriosclerotic peripheral vascular disease
See under AS.
(see AOD, ASCVD, ASHD, ASPVD, PVD)

ASS
Acute spinal stenosis
Acutely presenting narrowing of the spinal canal compromising the spinal cord.

AST
Aspartate amino transferase/aspartate transaminase
Enzyme present in liver and heart. A raised serum level indicates disease of either of these organs. This enzyme was formerly called glutamic oxaloacetic transaminase.
SGOT

ASVS
Arterial stimulation and venous sampling
Pancreatic and/or hepatic venous blood
sampling following a pancreatic arterial
injection of secretagogue for islet-cell tumours.

ATB
Antibiotic
See under AB.

ATCL
Adult T-cell lymphoma/leukaemia
Malignancies affecting T lymphocyte cell lines.
ATLL

ATG
Antithymocyte globulin
Type of intravenous (IV) immunosuppressive
therapy.

ATLL
Adult T-cell lymphoma/leukaemia
See under ATCL.

ATLS
Advanced trauma life support
American system of emergency initial
management of the trauma patient.

ATM
Asynchronous transfer mode
Very fast (155 Mbits/s) high bandwidth
network using a switching technique, ideal for
holding telemedicine conferences over long
distances.

ATN
Acute tubular necrosis
Renal tubular dysfunction resulting from
ischaemia. Cause of renal failure.
(*see ARF, CRF, RF*)

ATP
Adenosine triphosphate
Nucleotide energy source for metabolic
reactions.
(*see ADP*)

Atyp.
Atypical
Not conforming to type; uncharacteristic,
e.g. atypical pneumonia.

195m Au
Gold-195m
Radionuclide used in nuclear medicine for
angiocardiography.

AUA
Asymptomatic urinary abnormalities
Mild degree of microscopic haematuria or
pyuria, or small quantities of casts or protein in
the urine of patients who do not exhibit
symptoms of renal disease.
(*see ABU*)

Auto-BMT
Autologous bone marrow transplantation
Engraftment of patient's own bone marrow
back into his/her body after irradiation/other
immunosuppressive treatment to the patient
and graft.
(*see allo-BMT*)

AUV
Anterior urethral valves
Obstructive mucosal folds arising from the
anterior wall of the distal urethra. Rarer
congenital anomaly than posterior urethral
valves (PUV).

AV
Aortic valve
Heart valve between the left ventricle and the
aorta.
(*see AVR*)

AV
Arterio-venous
Connecting an artery and a vein, or
comprising arterial and venous elements.

AV
Atrio-ventricular
Connecting or related to these cardiac
chambers.

AVCx
Atrioventricular circumflex branch
Terminal branch of the left main-stem
coronary artery.

AVD
Aortic valve disease
Disordered performance of the cardiac aortic
valve. Can have numerous different causes.

AVF
Arteriovenous fistula
Abnormal connection between an artery and a
vein, it may result from malformation, tumour,
trauma or be artificially fashioned to give
access for haemodialysis.

aVF
Augmented volt foot
Electrocardiogram (ECG) lead giving
information on the electrical axis of the heart
and assisting in the localization of any ischaemic
changes in the inferior part of the heart.

AVH
Acute viral hepatitis
Acutely presenting viral infection of the liver.

AVHD
Acquired valvular heart disease
Disorders of cardiac valves that are not
congenital in nature.
(see CHD)

aVL
Augmented volt left
Electrocardiogram (ECG) lead giving
information on the electrical axis of the heart
and assisting in the localization of any ischaemic
changes in the left side of the heart.

AVM
Arteriovenous malformation
Congenital vascular lesion with arterial and
venous components.

AVN
Atrioventricular node
Specialized tissue lying between the atrial and
ventricular cardiac chambers which regulates
conduction of the cardiac cycle.

AVN
Atrioventricular node artery
Branch of the right coronary artery.

AVN
Avascular necrosis
See under AN.

AVNRT
AV node re-entry tachycardia
Type of cardiac dysrhythmia.
(see AVRT)

AVP
Arginine vasopressin
See under ADH.
(see DI)

AVR
Aortic valve replacement / repair
Surgical replacement or repair of the aortic
valve.
(see AV)

aVR
Augmented volt right
Electrocardiogram (ECG) lead giving
information on the electrical axis of the heart
and assisting in the localization of any
ischaemic changes in the right side of the
heart.

AVRT
Atrioventricular re-entry tachycardia
Cardiac dysrhythmia.
(see AVNRT)

AVS
Aortic valve stenosis
See under AS.

AWOL
Absent without leave

AxD
Axillary dissection
Surgical exploration of axilla for lymph nodes
during mastectomy to assist in staging breast
carcinoma.

AXR
Abdominal X-ray
Plain abdominal radiograph.
PAF
(see KUB)

Az
**Area under receiver–operator characteristic
curve**
Measure of test accuracy in receiver–operator
characteristic analysis (ROC analysis).

AZT
Azidothymidine (Zidovudine)
Drug which inhibits the human
immunodeficiency virus (HIV) in the
treatment of infected patients, whether
symptomatic or asymptomatic.
ZDV
(see AIDS)

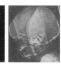

β-blocker
Beta-blocker
Member of a group of drugs acting on β-adrenergic receptors, slowing and reducing cardiac contractility (*inter alia*). Used commonly in angina and hypertension.

β⁺ decay
Beta plus decay
Form of radioactive decay more usually known as positron decay. Occurs in neutron-poor nuclides when a proton is transformed into a neutron and a positron is emitted. Used in positron emission tomography (PET).
β^+ emission

β⁻ decay
Beta minus decay
Form of radioactive decay. Occurs in neutron-rich nuclides when a neutron is transformed into a proton and an electron is emitted from the nucleus.
β^- emission

β⁺ emission
Beta plus emission
See under β^+ decay.

β⁻ emission
Beta minus emission
See under β^- decay.

β-HCG
Beta-human chorionic gonadotrophin
Hormone produced by a fertilized ovum, the presence of which may be used to confirm pregnancy. Also produced by malignant germ-cell tumours.
B-HCG, HCG

β-LPH
Beta lipotrophin
Anterior pituitary hormone secreted in response to corticotrophin-releasing factor (CRF).

β-MSH
Beta melanocyte stimulating hormone
Peptide produced from the precursor β-lipotrophin (β-LPH) in melantrophs of the pituitary pars intermedia.
(*see α-MSH, γ-MSH*)

β particle
Beta particle
Electron or positron emitted during beta decay.
(*see β^+ decay, β^- decay*)

β radiation
Beta radiation
Stream of beta particles (β particles).
β ray
(*see β particle*)

B
Bucky factor
Measure of the total quantity of radiation absorbed from an X-ray beam by a grid.
B = incident radiation / transmitted radiation.

B
Byte
8 bit data element.

B
Minimal detectable blurring
Minimum amount of detectable blurring of an object within the plane of cut in conventional tomography.

B₀
The main constant magnetic field of a magnetic resonance (MR) scanner.
H_0 (obsolete)

B₁
The induced field in magnetic resonance imaging (MRI).
H_1 (obsolete)

Ba
Barium
Element used as an enteric contrast medium in gastrointestinal (GI) radiology.
(*see BaE, BaFT, BaS, BE, BM, DCBE*)
Ba^{2+}

Ba²⁺
See under Ba.

BaE
Barium enema
Contrast examination of lower gastrointestinal tract, using barium as the contrast medium.
BE
(*see BaFT, BaS, BM, DCBE*)

BAER
Brainstem auditory evoked responses
Study of brain activity in response to auditory stimuli, using scalp electrodes.

BAFT

Barium follow-through
Contrast examination of the small bowel using oral contrast medium.
(*see Ba, BaE, BaS, BE, BM, DCBE*)

BAI

Basilar artery insufficiency
Hypoperfusion of the brain's basilar artery.

BAL

British anti-Lewisite (dimercaprol)
Drug used as an antidote in heavy metal poisoning.

BAL

Bronchoalveolar lavage
The introduction of fluid into the bronchi and alveoli at bronchoscopy for diagnostic or therapeutic purposes.
(*see BALF*)

BALF

Bronchoalveolar lavage fluid
Solution introduced through, and sampled by a bronchoscope to help in the diagnosis of pulmonary disease.
(*see BAL*)

BaS

Barium swallow
Contrast imaging of the pharynx and oesophagus.
(*see Ba, BaE, BaFT, BE, BM, DCBE*)

BASCHD

Bronchiectasis, asbestosis, scleroderma and other connective tissue diseases, cryptogenic fibrosing alveolitis, Hammon-Rich, drugs
Causes of interstitial lung fibrosis occurring predominantly in the lower zones of a chest radiograph (CXR).

Baud rate

Baudot rate
= one bit per second. Unit used for data transmission over a serial line.

BB

Blood bank
Department handling blood products.
Bld Bnk

BB

Breakthrough bleeding
Abnormal vaginal blood loss between menses, associated with hormonal imbalance and oral contraceptive use.
BTB

BBB

Blood–brain barrier
Anatomico-physiological separation between blood and cerebrospinal fluid (CSF).

BBS

Bulletin board system
Small, freely accessible database in which computer users can share information and programs with one another.

BC

Biliary colic
Pain caused by obstruction of the cystic duct or common bile duct, usually by a stone (calculus).

BC

Blood culture
Microbiological growth from a blood sample, relevant in suspected septicaemia.
BLC

BCC

Basal cell carcinoma
Malignant tumour of skin caused by excessive ultraviolet light.
BCE
(*see SSC*)

B cell

Bursa-equivalent cell
Lymphocyte derived from bone marrow; involved in antibody production.

BCE

Basal cell epithelioma
See under BCC.

BCG

Bacille Calmette–Guérin
Vaccine against tuberculosis (TB).

BCNU

N,N-*bis*(2-chloroethyl)-N-Nitrosurea
Carmustine: an antineoplastic agent.

BCR

British comparative ratio
Laboratory test for monitoring blood clotting, especially in patients on warfarin. Ratio of patient's prothrombin time (PT) to a control value.
INR

BCS

Budd–Chiari syndrome
Veno-occlusive disease (VOD) of the hepatic venous system, often presenting with a classic triad of symptoms: abdominal pain, hepatomegaly and ascites.

B&D
Bondage and discipline
Variant sexual behaviour which may be associated with unusual trauma.
(*see AC-DC, SM*)

bd
Bis in die
Twice a day.

BDE
Bile duct exploration
Surgical/endoscopic examination of the biliary tree.

BDL
Bile duct ligation
Surgical tying of the main extrahepatic biliary duct.

BDR
Background diabetic retinopathy
Non-proliferative changes in the retina of a diabetic patient.

BE
Bacterial endocarditis
Infection of the endothelium lining the heart, commonly in relation to an abnormal or prosthetic heart valve.
(*see ABE, SBE*)
IE

BE
Barium enema
See under BaE.
(*see Ba, BaFT, BaS, BM, DCBE, SCBE*)

BE
Base excess
Concentration of base in whole blood; can be used as a biochemical guide to the clinical acid–base status.

BFL
Bird fancier's lung
Hypersensitivity pneumonitis triggered by exposure to bird protein allergens.

BFS
Blood fasting sugar
Glucose measurement during fasting.

BG
Blood glucose
Serum glucose estimation.

BH
Braxton–Hicks contractions
Normal, low-intensity contractions of the uterus occurring after 30 weeks' gestation.

B-HCG
Beta-human chorionic gonadotrophin
See under β-HCG.
HCG

BHL
Bilateral hilar lymphadenopathy
Enlargement of the hilar lymph nodes in both lungs. Many possible causes but classically associated with sarcoidosis.

BHR
Bronchial hyper-reactivity
Increased responsiveness of airways to non-specific irritants. Occurs in extrinsic and intrinsic asthma.

BID
Brought in dead
Descriptive term of the state of a patient on arrival at the hospital.
DOA

BIH
Benign intracranial hypertension
Syndrome consisting of papilloedema with no demonstrable mass lesion and no increase in ventricular size.

BIN
tt-butylisonitrile
Tracer labelled with ^{99m}Technetium (^{99m}Tc) used in nuclear medicine for imaging myocardium and parathyroids.
HMIBI, MIBI

BIP
Biparietal diameter
Assessment of gestational age by ultrasound measurement of the fetal head in transverse section.
BPD

BIR
British Institute of Radiology
One of two official British radiological/oncological bodies. Members also include physicists and radiographers.
(*see RCR*)

Bit / bit
Binary digit
Smallest unit of memory in a computer. Can take values of zero or one, or be a switch set to on or off.

BJ
Biceps jerk
Involuntary contraction of biceps brachii muscles in response to sudden passive stretching of its tendon.

BJP
Bence–Jones protein
Free monoclonal light chains or fragments present in the urine of patients with myeloma.

BJR
British Journal of Radiology
Monthly peer-reviewed journal of the British Institute of Radiology (BIR).

BKA
Below-knee amputation
(see AKA)

BKG
Background

BKWP
Below-knee walking plaster
Plaster of Paris cast stabilizing and immobilizing the lower limb..

Bl
Bladder

BLC
Blood culture
See under BC.

Bld Bnk (US: BB)
Blood bank
See under BB.

Bleo.
Bleomycin
Anti-mitotic drug, also used for pleurodesis.

BLS
Basic life support
Essential initial life saving measures: airway, breathing, circulation (ABC).
(see AR, CPR, ECM)

BM
Barium meal
Contrast examination of oesophagus, stomach and duodenum, using barium as the contrast medium.
(see Ba, BaE, BaFT, BaS, DCBE)

BMA
British Medical Association
Organization representing the British medical profession.
(see BMJ)

BMD
Bone mineral density
Density of bone.
(see DEXA, DXA, HRT)

BMI
Body mass index
Weight in kilograms divided by square of height in metres; allows quantitation of obesity (normally taken to be <30 kg/m^2).

BMJ
British Medical Journal
Weekly peer-reviewed journal of the British Medical Association.
Br. Med. J

B-MODE
Brightness mode
Ultrasound technique displaying ultrasound echoes from a slice of tissue.

BMR
Basal metabolic rate
Measure of oxygen consumption at rest.

BM-stix
Blood monitoring sticks
Proprietary diagnostic 'stick' test for rapid monitoring of capillary glucose levels, using a pin-prick sample of blood.

BMT
Bone marrow transplantation/transplant
The introduction of bone marrow cells into an individual as treatment for a haematological disorder or to replace native cells destroyed by therapy.

BMUS
British Medical Ultrasound Society
Main scientific body for ultrasound in the UK.

BMZ
Basement membrane zone
Area described by optical microscopy between an epithelial cell layer and the underlying connective tissue.

BNF
British National Formulary
Compendium of drugs available in Great Britain for prescription by licensed practitioners.

BNO
Bladder neck obstruction
Urinary tract outflow obstruction at the level of the bladder neck.

BNO
Bowels not open
Nursing or medical note.

BO
Body odour
Unpleasant smell emanating from human body. Usually due to poor personal hygiene.

BO
Bowels open
Nursing or medical note.

BO
Bronchiotitis obliterans
A pathological diagnosis where bronchioles are obstructed by organizing exudate, granulation tissue and fibrosis. May result from a variety of initiating stimuli.
(see COP)

B₀
Magnetic field
The constant applied magnetic field in magnetic resonance.

BOLD
Blood oxygen level dependent (contrast)
A magnetic resonance gradient echo (GE) technique using blood as an endogenous contrast medium.

BOOP
Bronchiolitis obliterans with organizing pneumonia
Bronchiolitis with extension of granulation tissue distally into the alveoli. Usually responds to steroids.
(see COP)

BP
Blood pressure
Systemic arterial pressure of blood, usually measured with a sphygmomanometer and recorded during both the systolic and diastolic phases of the cardiac cycle.
ABP
(see HT)

BP
Breech presentation
The presenting fetal part is the breech (hindquarters).

BPD
Biparietal diameter
See under BIP.

BPH
Benign prostatic hyperplasia
Non-malignant enlargement of the prostate gland.

bpm
Beats per minute
Refers to the heart rate.

bps
Bits per second
Measurement of transmission speed across a network.

BPS
Biophysical profile score
Assessment of fetal well-being recorded numerically according to predefined criteria.

BPV
Benign positional vertigo
Rotatory sensation precipitated by the adoption of certain positions.

BPV
Bioprosthetic valve
Animal-derived arificial heart valve (porcine).

Bq
Becquerel
SI unit of the rate of radioactive decay.
1 Bq = 1 disintegration per second.
(see Ci, GBq, kBq, MBq, mCi, microCi)

Br
Bromine
Waste product of X-ray film processing resulting from the reduction of silver bromide (AgBr).

BRBPR (US)
Bright red blood per rectum
The passage of fresh blood from the anus.

BREASTS
Bronchopulmonary aspergillosis, radiotherapy, extrinsic allergic alveolitis, ankylosing spondylitis, sarcoidosis, tuberculosis, silicosis
Radiological causes of upper zone fibrotic lung changes on chest x-ray (CXR).
TRASHES

BRH
Benign recurrent haematuria
Repeated episodes of passing blood in the urine for which no pathological cause is found.

BRH
Bureau of Radiological Health
US Federal authority concerned with radiation protection.

Br. Med. J.
British Medical Journal
See under BMJ.

Bronch.
Bronchoscopy
Endoscopic examination of the trachea and airways.

BS
Bachelor of Surgery
Basic medical qualification.

BS
Blood sugar
Quantity of glucose in the blood expressed as mmol/l.

BS
Bowel sounds
Noise of gut peristalsis. Clinical sign particularly relevant in the acute abdomen and in post-operative assessment.

BS
Breath sounds
Sounds heard with a stethoscope (or ear) during the respiratory cycle.

BSA
Body surface area
Assessed in a patient using a height /weight nomogram.

BSc
Bachelor of Science
Basic scientific degree.

BSE
Breast self-examination
Technique of self-palpation of breasts, undertaken to detect early breast lumps.

BSIR
British Society of Interventional Radiology
Society concerned with the teaching and practice of interventional radiology in the UK.
(see APSCVIR, CIRSE, JIR, JSAIR, SCVIR, WAIS)

BSO
Bilateral salpingo-oophorectomy
Surgical removal of both Fallopian tubes and ovaries.

B–S Valve
Bjork–Shiley valve
Tilting disc prosthetic heart valve.

BT
Bladder tumour
Neoplastic bladder growth.

BT
Bleeding time
Parameter used in the assessment of coagulation status.

BTB
Breakthrough bleeding
See under BB.

BTD
Biliary tract disease
Any condition affecting the intra- or extra-hepatic biliary system.

BTS
Brady–tachy syndrome
Cardiac conduction defect of the sinuatrial node, causing brady/tachy–arrhythmias.
(see SSS)

BT shunt
Blalock–Taussig shunt
Surgical treatment for Fallot's tetralogy. Anastomosis between a subclavian artery and a pulmonary artery.
(see CHD, FT)

BTx
Blood transfusion
Intravenous (IV) administration of donor cross-matched blood (XM) to treat anaemia/blood loss.

BU
Burns unit
Specialized department for the care of burns.

BUN
Blood urea nitrogen
US term for urea concentration.
U, Ur

BV
Basilic vein
Arm vein in medial antecubital fossa which drains into the axillary vein.

BV
Blood vessel
Artery, vein or capillary.

BVH
Biventricular hypertrophy
Wall enlargement of both cardiac ventricles.

BW
Birth weight
Weight of new-born infant.
Bwt

BW
Bladder washout
Irrigation of the bladder via a catheter.

BW
Body weight
A person's weight.
Bwt

Bwt
Birth weight
See under BW.

Bwt
Body weight
See under BW.

Bx
Biopsy
Removal and examination of body tissue.

C-1, C-2, C-3, ... – C-9

Complement factor 1, Complement factor 2, ...
Nine protein compounds of the complement system. Part of the body's immune system critical for opsonization in preparation for phagocytosis.

C-14, 14-C

Carbon-14, ^{14}C
Radionuclide used in nuclear medicine for breath tests to assess absorption from the small intestine.

c

calorie
Non SI unit of energy (E). 1c = 4.1855 Joule (J). One Calorie (i.e. 1 Kilocalorie) = 1000 calories; this latter unit is used to indicate the energy value of foods.
(see C, SI unit)

c

Canine
Pointed tooth lying between the incisors and the pre-molars.

c̄

Cum
Latin for 'with'.

c

Speed of light
Velocity (v) at which electromagnetic waves (EM waves) travel. c = 3×10^8 m/s.
(see γrays)

C

Calorie
1 Calorie = 1 kilocalorie (= 1000 calories). Non SI unit of energy. Used to indicate the energy value of foods.
(see c, J)

C

Carbon
The element carbon.

C

Celsius, centigrade
Non SI unit of temperature (T). C° = ⁵⁄₉(F°–32); C° = K°–273.15.
(see F, K)

C

Cervical nerve root
Used with a number 1–8 to define the root level.

C

Cervical vertebra
Used with a number 1–7 to define the particular vertebra.

C

Contrast
1. Radiographic contrast: difference in density between two different parts of a radiograph.
2. Subject contrast: difference in X-ray intensities (I) transmitted through two different parts of a body.

^{14}C

Carbon-14
See under C-14.

C

Coulomb
SI unit of charge.

C

Count
Radioactive disintegration recorded by a detector system.
(see cpc)

^{125}Ca

A radiolabelled non-specific tumour marker for colorectal malignancy.

Ca²⁺-blocker

Calcium channel blocker
One of a group of drugs inhibiting cellular calcium channels, producing vasodilatation. Commonly used in angina, hypertension, and heart failure.

Ca²⁺

Calcium
Ca

Ca

Calcium
Ca²⁺

Ca.

Cancer
Malignant neoplasm.

Ca.

Carcinoma
Malignant growth of epithelial cells.

CA

Candida albicans
Fungal micro-organism causing generalized and local infections (thrush) particularly of mucous membranes (mouth, vagina); infective agent common in immunosuppressed patients.

CA

Cardiac arrest
Sudden loss of cardiac output owing to catastrophic arrhythmia.
(see EMD)

CA

Coeliac axis
Vascular trunk arising from the aorta (T12/L1), giving rise to the common hepatic, splenic and left gastric arteries.

CA

Coronary artery
One of two principal blood vessels supplying the heart.

CAAT

Computer assisted axial tomography
Imaging modality using X-rays to produce a cross-sectional scan of a patient. CT is now the common term.
CAT, CT

CAB

Coronary artery bypass
Operation to improve the blood supply to the myocardium.
CABG

CABG

Coronary artery bypass graft
See under CAB.

CAD

Computer aided design
Computer program used to create precisely scaled technical drawing.

CAD

Computer aided diagnosis
Computer algorithm designed to detect specific diagnostic features, e.g. in a radiographic image.

CAD

Coronary artery disease
Atherosclerotic changes in the coronary arteries.
(see IHD)

CAH

Chronic active hepatitis
Disease of diverse aetiology, characterized by continuing hepatic inflammation, necrosis and fibrosis which may lead to cirrhosis, liver failure and death.

CAH

Congenital adrenal hyperplasia
Deficiency of an adrenal cortical enzyme involved in the synthesis of cortisol. This results in the increased production of androgens from steroid precursors owing to increased ACTH production.

CAL

Chronic airflow limitation
Pulmonary disease causing a progressive, predominantly expiratory, limitation of the airflow; includes emphysema, bronchitis and chronic asthma.
COAD, COAL, COLD, COPD

CAM

Cystic adenomatoid malformation
Benign lung abnormality, seen in neonates.

cAMP

Cyclic adenosine monophosphate
A nucleotide activating enzyme system within the cell.

CAMs

Cell adhesion molecules
Molecular entities responsible for cells sticking to one another or to other surfaces.

CAPD

Continuous ambulatory peritoneal dialysis
Renal replacement therapy allowing excretion of metabolic waste into the peritoneal fluid which is exchanged regularly via a permanent catheter. Allows patient to remain mobile.
(see APD, CCPD, IPD)

CAR

Computer Assisted Radiology
Organization based in Europe concerned with computer and communication technologies applied to digital imaging in medical diagnosis and therapy.

C Arm

C-shaped arm
Shaped gantry supporting an X-ray tube, permitting its movement around the longitudinal axis of the examination couch.

Cas.

Casualty (from latin: *casu* – by chance)
Casualty department (accident and emergency department).
A & E

CAT

Computer assisted tomography
See under CAAT.
CT

CAT scan

Computer assisted tomography scan
Image or set of images obtained with a computer assisted tomography scanner. (CAT scanner).
CT Scan
(*see* CT)

CAT scanner

Computer assisted tomography scanner
Computer assisted tomography (CAT) machine.
CT Scanner
(*see* CT)

Cauc. (US: WM/WF: white male/white female)

Caucasian
White (racial description).

CAVG

Coronary artery vein graft(s)
Operation to improve the blood supply to the myocardium using venous grafts.
(*see* CAB, CABG)

CAVHD

Continuous arteriovenous haemodialysis
Renal replacement therapy involving dialysis of blood removed from and returned to the body through a specially fashioned AV fistula.

CaWO$_4$

Calcium tungstate
Original phosphor used in X-ray intensifier screens. Not commonly found in modern X-ray equipment.

CB

Conus branch
First branch of the right coronary artery.

CBC

Complete blood count
Quantitation of the major blood components.
FBC

CBD

Common bile duct
Main vessel draining bile from the liver and gall bladder into the duodenum.
(*see* CD)

CBF

Cerebral blood flow
Blood flowing through the brain.

CBT

Computer based training
Learning programme conducted on a computer screen.
(*see* GUI)

CBV

Cerebral blood volume
The volume of blood in the vessels of the brain.

cc

Copies circulated
Precedes list of names of people to whom a copy of the document has been sent.

CC

Cholecalciferol, Vitamin D
Vitamin formed in the skin which is important in calcium metabolism. Its deficiency causes osteomalacia in adults or rickets in children.

CC

Craniocaudad
Refers to a direction of the beam in radiography, in this case directed from head to feet.

CC

Creatinine clearance
A measure of glomerular filtration rate (GFR), which is the volume of fluid filtered by glomeruli per minute. An indicator of renal function.

$$CC = \frac{[creatine]\ urine}{[creatine]\ plasma} \times urine\ flow\ rate$$

CC

Crohn's colitis
Chronic inflammatory disease of the colon; causes abdominal pain, fever and diarrhoea, may also affect the entire gastro-intestinal tract.
(*see* CD)

CCA

Common carotid artery
Branch of the aorta which supplies parts of the brain, head and neck (one of two such arteries).

CCD

Charged-coupled device
Semiconductor chip which behaves as if consisting of multiple arrays of small internal capacitors from which a digital signal is produced by the application of an electrical signal.

CCF

Congestive cardiac failure
Inability of the heart to pump blood efficiently resulting in shortness of breath and fluid accumulation. It implies right ventricular failure secondary to left ventricular failure.
CHF
(see HF, LVF, RVF)

CCITT

Comité Consultatif Internationale Télégraphique et Téléphonique
International organization that devises and proposes recommendations for international telecommunications.

CCK

Cholecystokinin
Gut hormone produced by the amine precursor uptake and decarboxylation (APUD) cells of the upper small bowel. It causes gallbladder contraction, pancreatic enzyme secretion and increased gut motility.

CCL

Communications control language
Language used to write connect sequence files for computers.

CCPD

Continuous cyclic peritoneal dialysis
A variant of continuous ambulatory peritoneal dialysis (CAPD) renal replacement therapy performed at night during sleep. Automatic cycler equipment dispenses and drains the dialysis fluid.
(see APD, IPD)

CCT

Contrast enhanced computed tomography
Computed tomography (CT) during which a bolus of intravenous contrast medium is injected to enhance vessels and vascular tissue.
CECT
(see NECT)

CCU

Coronary care unit
Specially equipped ward for the intensive care of cardiac patients.

CD

Coeliac disease
Gluten intolerance causing intestinal villous atrophy and malabsorption.

CD

Colour Doppler
Ultrasound technique combining a cross-sectional image with a colour representation of the direction and speed of flow within vessels.
CDI, CFDU, CFI

CD

Common (hepatic) duct
Intrahepatic portion of the main bile duct before it is joined by the cystic duct to form the common bile duct (CBD).
CHD

CD

Conjugata diagonalis
Diameter of the pelvic inlet

CD

Controlled drugs
Medication (usually opiate) subject to the prescription requirements of the Misuse of Drugs Regulations 1985.

CD

Compact disc
Digital optical medium for storing data. Type of optical disc.

CD

Crohn's disease
Chronic inflammatory disease commonly affecting the terminal ileum, but which can also result in discontinuous involvement of the whole gastro-intestinal tract. May be associated with extraintestinal manifestations.
(see CC)

CD4

Cluster of differentiation antigen (T4-helper cell)
Serum quantitation of the circulating population of 'helper' T-lymphocytes (T_h); intimately involved in immune defence. Low count in acquired immunodeficiency syndrome (AIDS).

CDE

Colour Doppler energy imaging
Ultrasound technique combining a cross-sectional image with a colour representation of flow within vessels. Very sensitive to slow flow; contains no information about flow direction or speed.

C. difficile

Clostridium difficile
Gram positive bacterium; major cause of colitis
in antibiotic-associated diarrhoea.
(*see AAC, AAPC, PMC*)

CDH

Congenital dislocation of the hip
Hip joint instability in neonates with shallow
acetabulum and lax joint. May become
permanent if untreated.

CDI

Colour Doppler imaging
See under CD.
CFDU, CFI

CD-ROM

Compact disc – read only memory
Type of optical disc whose data can be read
but not rewritten.

CE

Carotid endarterectomy
Surgical procedure to relieve carotid artery
stenosis by the removal of occlusive material.

CEA

Carcinoembryonic antigen
A serological marker for colorectal cancer, but
which has poor specificity.

CEC

Central echo complex
Increased reflectivity in the centre of the
kidney caused by fat.

CECT

Contrast enhanced computed tomography
See under CCT.
(*see NECT*)

CEP

Congenital erythropoietic porphyria
Recessively-inherited, rare defect of porphyrin
metabolism causing chronic photosensitivity
with mutilating skin lesions and haemolytic
anaemia.

cf

Confer
Latin for: refer to.

CF

Cystic fibrosis
Autosomal-recessive, inherited condition
causing chronic suppurative lung disease,
pancreatic insufficiency, biliary cirrhosis and
male infertility.

CFA

Cryptogenic fibrosing alveolitis
Progressive pulmonary fibrosis of unknown
cause.
FA, IPF, UIP

CFDU

Colour flow Doppler ultrasound
See under CD.
CDI, CFI

CFI

Colour flow imaging
See under CD.
CDI, CFDU

CFT

Complement fixation test
Test used in immunology.

CGA

Colour graphics adaptor
An early standard for personal computer
graphics. Unsatisfactory for image-processing
applications.

CGN

Chronic glomerulonephritis
Glomerulonephritis (GN) characterized by
persistent urinary abnormalities and slowly
progressive impairment of renal function.
(*see CRF, ESRF, RF, RPGN*)

CHA

Common hepatic artery
Branch of the coeliac axis, supplying the liver
and gallbladder and giving rise to the
gastroduodenal artery.

CHAD

Cold haemagglutinin disease
A chronic intravascular haemolytic anaemia
which is exacerbated by a cold environment.

CHB

Complete heart block
Failure of conduction of cardiac atrial
electrical activity to the ventricles.
A condition commonly requiring pacing.
TAVB

CHD

Common hepatic duct
See under CD.
(*see CBD*)

CHD

Congenital heart disease
A spectrum of developmental abnormalities affecting the heart.
(see ASD, AVHD, BT Shunt, C of A, ECD, FT, HLHS, IAA, KSS, TA, TAPVC, TGA, TGV, UAPA)

CHD

Coronary heart disease
Reduced heart muscle perfusion, usually due to atherosclerosis. Causes angina and may result in infarction.
IHD
(see MI)

CHE

Chemoembolization
Technique in interventional radiology combining local intra-arterial chemotherapy of a tumour with embolization of its feeding vessel(s).

chemo.

Chemotherapy
Medical treatment of malignant tumours using one or more different cytotoxic drugs.
CMT

CHESS

Chemical shift selective
Magnetic resonance radio-frequency pulse sequence which allows differentiation of the chemical components of tissues.

CHF

Congenital hepatic fibrosis
Congenital liver disorders.

CHF

Congestive heart failure
See under CCF.
(see HF, LVF, RVF)

C₂H₅OH

Ethanol
Ethyl alcohol.
EtOH
(see AOB, DTs)

Ci

Curie
Historic unit of the rate of radioactive decay. Has been replaced by the Becquerel (Bq).
$1 \text{ Ci} = 3.7 \times 10^{10}$ Bq.
(see kBq, Mbq, μCi, mCi)

CI

Cardiac index
Cardiac output expressed as a fraction of body surface area.

CI

Confidence interval
Measure of the accuracy of an estimated value in statistics.

CI

Contraindication
Factor making it imprudent to pursue a certain course of action.

CIC

Clean intermittent catheterization
Treatment for incontinence using regular drainage of the bladder with a reusable catheter.

CIDP

Chronic inflammatory demyelinating polyneuropathy
Group of chronic progressive or relapsing inflammatory demyelinating peripheral neuropathies mostly affecting the sensory nerves and associated with elevated paraproteins.

CIE

Counter-current immune electrophoresis
Technique in immunology.

CIN

Cervical intra-epithelial neoplasm
Non-invasive, abnormal changes in cells of the cervix regarded as precursors of malignancy.

CIRSE

Cardiovascular and Interventional Radiological Society of Europe
Official European radiological body concerned with cardiovascular and interventional radiology.
(see APSCVIR, BSIR, CVIR, JSAIR, SCVIR, WAIS)

CIS

Carcinoma in situ
Minute, intra-epithelial malignant focus, often considered to be a precancerous state.
TIS

CJD
Creutzfeldt–Jacob disease
Fatal degenerative disease of the central
nervous system with rapidly evolving dementia
and myoclonus. It is caused by infection with a
slow virus.
JCD, JKD, KJD

CK
Creatine (phospho) kinase
Enzyme found in heart muscle, brain and
skeletal muscle. Elevated serum levels indicate
damage to any of these tissues.
CPK

CKMB
Creatine kinase myocardial bound
Isoenzyme fraction specific for cardiac damage.
(see CK, CPK)

Cl⁻
Chloride
Principal extracellular anion.

Clin. Rad.
Clinical Radiology
Monthly peer-reviewed journal of Royal
College of Radiologists (RCR).
Clin. Radiol.

Clin. Radiol.
Clinical Radiology
See under Clin. Rad.

CLIP
Corticotrophin-like intermediate lobe peptide
Peptide produced from the presursor
adrenocorticotrophic hormone (ACTH) in
melanotrophs of the pituitary pars intermedia.

CLL
Chronic lymphocytic/lymphatic leukaemia
Neoplastic proliferation of differentiated
lymphoid white blood cells which infiltrate
bone marrow, spleen and lymph nodes.

CM
Contrast medium
Agent used in imaging to enhance
visualization of anatomical structures.

cm
Centimetre
10^{-2} metre (m).

CMC
Computer mediated communication
Dissemination of information using a
computer, often over the Internet.

CMCJ
Carpometacarpal joint
One of several synovial joints between the
wrist bones and the metacarpals.

CMD
Congenital muscular dystrophy
A muscle disease of progressive weakness
dating from birth.

CME
Continuing medical education
System for ensuring continuity of education
after qualification. Educational credits are
awarded by the appropriate bodies for
attending meetings, etc.

CMG
Cystometrogram
Investigation of bladder function.

CML
Chronic myeloid (myelogenous) leukaemia
A myeloproliferative disorder caused by
neoplastic proliferation of bone marrow cells,
often affecting red and white cells and platelets
and characterized by massive splenomegaly.

CMML
Chronic myelomonocytic leukaemia
Type of chronic myeloid leukaemia (CML).

CMT
Chemotherapy
See under chemo.

CMV
Cytomegalovirus
Herpes virus family member causing severe
birth defects and a wide spectrum of diseases in
adults, especially immunocompromised
individuals.

CNI, CN1; 1
First cranial nerve (olfactory)

CNII, CN2; II
Second cranial nerve (optic)

CNIII, CN3; III
Third cranial nerve (oculomotor)

CNIV, CN4; IV
Fourth cranial nerve (trochlear)

CNV, CN5; V
Fifth cranial nerve (trigeminal)

CNVI, CN6; VI
Sixth cranial nerve (abducens)

CNVII, CN7; VII

Seventh cranial nerve (facial)

CNVIII, CN8; VIII

Eighth cranial nerve (vestibulocochlear)

CNIX, CN9; IX

Ninth cranial nerve (glossopharyngeal)

CNX, CN10; X

Tenth cranial nerve (vagus)

CNXI

Eleventh cranial nerve (accessory)
CN11; XI

CNXII

Twelfth cranial nerve (hypoglossal)
CN12; XII

CN

Cranial nerve
One of 12 nerves whose nuclei lie within the
pons, medulla or midbrain.
(see CNI – CNXII)

CNS

Central nervous system
Nervous tissue enclosed within meninges:
brain and spinal cord.

$^{14}CO_2$

Carbon dioxide-14
Carbon-14 (^{14}C) labelled carbon dioxide
(CO_2). Metabolic product used in breath tests
for malabsorption.

c/o

Complaining of
Main symptom which caused patient to
consult doctor.
p/c, PC

CO

Carbon monoxide
Gas which if inhaled binds avidly to
haemoglobin resulting in brain damage,
myocardial damage and death.

^{57}Co, 57-Co

Cobalt-57
Radionuclide used in nuclear medicine for
investigating vitamin B12 deficiency
(Schilling test).
(see ^{58}Co)

^{58}Co, 58-Co

Cobalt-58
Radionuclide used in nuclear medicine for
investigating vitamin B12 deficiency
(Schilling test).
(see ^{57}Co)

CO_2

Carbon dioxide
Gaseous waste product of metabolism in the
animal kingdom. Also used as intravenous (iv)
contrast medium for grey scale ultrasound
(US) and as an arterial contrast medium in
angiography.

COAD

Chronic obstructive airways disease
See under CAL.
COAL, COLD, COPD

COAL

Chronic obstructive air-flow limitation
See under CAL.
COAD, COLD, COPD

coarct.

Coarctation (of aorta)
Developmental obstruction of aorta distal to
the left subclavian artery (type A), between
the left subclavian and left carotid arteries,
or between the innominate and left carotid
arteries. The distal blood supply is
maintained through a patent ductus
arteriosus, which may constrict shortly
after birth.
C of A, IAA
(see Ao, CHD)

COC

Combined oral contraceptive
Cyclical hormone administration including
oestrogen, aimed at preventing ovulation.
COCP

COCP

Combined oral contraceptive pill
See under COC.

COD

Cause of death

C of A

Coarctation of aorta
See under coarct.

C of E
Church of England
Established protestant church in England.
(*see RC*)

COLD
Chronic obstructive lung disease
See under CAL.
COAL, COAD, COPD

Colles
Colles' fracture
Impacted fracture of distal radius with dorsal angulation of the distal fragment. Avulsion of the ulnar styloid may also occur.
(*see Smith's*)

com.(s)
Communication(s)
Instructions, usually written.

COM
Chronic otitis media
Chronic suppurative inflammation of the middle ear cavity, often with perforation of the ear drum.
(*see AOM, CSOM*)

Com. port
Communications port
Serial connection socket to connect a modem, mouse or printer to a computer.

COP
Cryptogenic organizing pneumonitis
Bronchiolitis with extension of granulation tissue distally into the alveoli. Usually responds to steroids.
(*see BOOP*)

COPD
Chronic obstructive pulmonary disease
See under CAL.
COAD, COAL, COLD

cos.
Cosine
Periodic mathematical function. Ratio of adjacent/hypotenuse sides of a triangle.

CP
Cephalic presentation
Vertex birth presentation: the fetal head is the lowermost part in the maternal pelvis.

CP
Cerebral palsy
Motor neurological deficit in children caused by hypoxic brain damage at birth.
ICP

CP
Chronic pancreatitis
Chronic inflammation of the pancreas, presenting as recurrent acute inflammation or persistent abdominal pain or malabsorption.

CP sequence
Carr–Purcell sequence
Magnetic resonance sequence of a 90 degree radiofrequency (RF) pulse followed by repeated 180 degree RF pulses to produce a train of spin echoes.

CPA
Cerebellopontine angle
Brain stem angle between cerebellum and pons where cranial nerves V, VI, VII, VIII exit.

CPAP
Continuous positive airways pressure
Ventilatory support method used in weaning from artificial ventilation.

CPD
Cephalo-pelvic disproportion
Term used in obstetric practice to indicate disproportion between fetal head and maternal pelvis.

CPDA
Citrate/phosphate/dextrose-adenine
An anticoagulant used in stored blood.

CPH
Chronic persistent hepatitis
Continuing hepatic inflammation following viral infection (usually B, and non-A, non-B). Usually non-progressive. Cirrhosis and liver failure are rare.

CPK
Creatine phosphokinase
See under CK.

CPMG sequence
Carr–Purcell–Meiboom–Gill sequence
Modification of the Carr–Purcell magnetic resonance sequence to reduce the accumulating effects of imperfections in the 180-degree pulse.

CPP

Cerebral perfusion pressure
Pressure of blood perfusing the brain. A value below 40–60 mmHg is considered to be detrimental to nerve cells.

CPPD

Calcium pyrophosphate dihydrate
Crystal which forms in joints causing a synovitis in pseudogout.

CPR

Cardiopulmonary resuscitation
Technique for resuscitating a patient after cardiorespiratory arrest. Involves external cardiac massage (ECM) and artificial ventilation.
(see ABC, AR, BLS)

cps

counts per second
Number of radioactive disintegrations recorded by a detector system per second.
(see Bq)

cps

Cycles per second
Number of cyclical occurrences every second.

CPS

Characters per second
Measure of printing speed for dot matrix printers.

CPU

Central processing unit
Computer hardware that manipulates data and controls the sequence of computer operations.

CQI

Continuous quality improvement
A statistical method of assessing performance.
(see TQM)

CR

Clinical remission (complete remission)
Treated disorder currently asymptomatic and showing no clinical evidence of active disease (e.g. malignant disease).

CR

Computed radiography
Modality using laser-read, photostimulable phosphor plates (PSP) to produce hard or soft copy digital radiographic images.
DLR, DR, PSL

Cr

Creatinine
Metabolite excreted from cells. The plasma level of creatinine is a measure of renal function.
Creat.

^{51}Cr

Chromium-51
Radionuclide used in nuclear medicine for measuring glomerular filtration rate (GFR).
51-Cr

CRAO

Central retinal artery occlusion
Blockage of the arterial blood vessel supplying the back of the eye, resulting in blindness.

CRAW

Computed radiography acquisition workstation
Unit which assimilates the digital image acquired by the computed radiography (CR) plate reader and sends it to a picture archiving and communications system (PACS).

Creat.

Creatinine
See under Cr.

CREST

Calcinosis, Raynaud's phenomenon, Oesophageal disorder, Sclerodactyly, Telangiectasia
Features associated with autoimmune connective tissue disease. CREST syndrome: variant of systemic sclerosis (SS) associated with an improved prognosis.

CRF

Chronic renal failure
Kidney impairment resulting from gradual destruction of the renal parenchyma.
RF
(see ARF, ATN, CGN, ESRF)

CRF

Corticotrophin releasing factor
Hormone produced by the hypothalamus, important in regulating the release of adrenocorticotrophic hormone (ACTH) from the pituitary.
CRH

CRH

Corticotrophin releasing hormone
See under CRF.

CRITOL

Capitellum, radial head, inner epicondyle, trochlea, olecranon, lateral epicondyle
Mnemonic for the order of radiographic appearance of epiphyses of the elbow.

CRL

Crown rump length
Ultrasound measurement of head–tail length to estimate fetal age.

CRP

C-reactive protein
Hepatic protein synthesised in the 'acute phase response', principally in inflammatory disorders.

CRT

Cadaveric renal transplant
Transplanted kidney from a dead donor.

CRT

Cathode ray tube
Vacuum tube for focusing a beam of electrodes to form a spot of light on a fluorescent screen.

CRVO

Central retinal vein occlusion
Obstruction of the principal vein draining the retina, usually resulting in blindness.

Cryoppt

Cryoprecipitate
Autoantibody which precipitates out of blood at low temperatures, thereby increasing its viscosity and resulting in the impairment of blood flow, especially through the peripheral capillaries of fingers, toes and nose.

C/S

Caesarian section
Operation to remove a baby directly from the uterus through the maternal abdominal wall.
CS

CS

Caesarian section
See under C/S.

CSDMS

Canadian Society of Diagnostic Medical Sonographers
Professional body of ultrasonographers, which publishes a quarterly newsletter: Interface.

CSF

Cerebrospinal fluid
Fluid bathing the brain and spinal cord.
Sp. fl.
(see BBB)

CSG

Cholecystogram
Imaging study of the opacified gall bladder.
(see AFM)

CSI

Chemical shift imaging
Magnetic resonance technique which provides spectral resolution coupled to a degree of spatial localization.

CsI

Caesium iodide
Phosphor commonly used for input fluorescent screens in modern image intensifiers (II).
(see (ZnCd)S)

CSMA/CD

Carrier sense multiple access/collision detection
A network protocol allowing only one device to transmit at a time (used on networks with bus topology).

CSMAP

Coeliac-superior mesenteric arterial portography
Imaging of the hepatic portal vein by the injection of contrast medium into the coeliac axis and superior mesenteric artery.

CSOM

Chronic suppurative otitis media
Chronic ear infection with purulent discharge.
(see AOM, COM)

CSSD

Central sterile supply department
Unit for storage, sterilization and distribution of sterile dressings, equipment, linen, etc.
CSSU
(see TSSD, TSSU)

CSSU

Central sterile supply unit
See under CSSD.

CST

Contractions stress test
Ultrasound monitoring of fetal heart rate during uterine contractions.

CT

Calcitonin
Potent hypocalcaemic hormone which acts in many ways as a physiological antagonist to parathyroid hormone. Secreted by thyroid C cells.

CT

Cardiothoracic ratio
Numerical value used to assess heart size radiologically. The transverse diameter of the heart is expressed as a percentage of the transverse diameter of the thorax. Should be less than 50% in adults.
CTR

CT

Computed tomography
See under CAAT.
CAT

CT scan

Computed tomography scan
1. Image or set of images obtained with a computed tomography scanner (CT scanner).
2. The procedure itself.
CAT scan

CT scanner

Computed tomography scanner
Computed tomography (CT) machine.
CT Scanner

CTAP

Computed tomography (during) arterial portography
Computed tomography (CT) during the intra-arterial (IA) injection of contrast medium into the splenic or superior mesenteric artery (SMA) through an angiography catheter.

CTG

Cardiotocogram (-graph)
Fetal heart rate monitor using Doppler ultrasound.
TG

CTR

Cardiothoracic ratio
See under CT.
CT

CTR

Carpal tunnel release
Surgical procedure for the treatment of carpal tunnel syndrome (CTS).

CTS

Carpal tunnel syndrome
Compression of the median nerve at the wrist causing pain, paraesthesia and muscle wasting.

CTX

Clinical trial exemption
Permission to administer an investigational agent to patients/volunteers under the specified conditions of a particular research study in a clinical setting.

Cu

Copper
Metal used for X-ray filtration, e.g. in CT.

CV

Cephalic vein
Superficial arm vein in the lateral antecubital fossa, which drains into the axillary vein.

CV

Conjugata vera
True conjugate; diameter of pelvic outlet.
CVO

CVA

Cerebrovascular accident
Acute neurological injury as a result of ischaemia or haemorrhage. A 'stroke', or apoplexy.

CVB

Chorionic villous biopsy
Sampling of placental material, usually via a transvaginal approach. Used in prenatal diagnosis of genetic disease.
CVS

CVIR

CardioVascular and Inteventional Radiology
Journal which is the official organ of the Cardiovasular and International Society of Europe and the Japanese Society of Angiography and Interventional Radiology.
(see CIRSE, JSAIR)

CVO

Conjugata vera obstetrica
See under CV.

CVP

Central venous pressure
The cardiac filling pressure. Usually measured through a catheter sited in one of the great central veins using a jugular or subclavian approach.
(see JVP)

CVS
Cardiovascular system
Heart and peripheral circulatory system.

CVS
Chorionic villous sampling
See under CVB.

CVVHD
Continuous veno–venous haemodialysis
Renal therapy involving the dialysis of blood
removed from and returned to the circulation
by the venous route.

CW
Continuous wave
1. In ultrasound: assessment of peripheral
blood vessel flow using a Doppler signal which
is continually emitted and received by the
probe.
2. In magnetic resonance: electromagnetic
field that oscillates sinusoidally with time.

CWP
Coal worker's pneumoconiosis
Lung parenchymal reaction to the deposition
of coal dust which may eventually result in
fibrosis.

Cx
Cervical
Pertaining to the neck, e.g. cervical spine.

Cx
Cervix
Uterine neck.

Cx
Complication

CXR
Chest X-ray
Radiograph of the thorax.

D

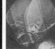

2-D
Two-dimensional
Refers to imaging modalities and images in radiology in which data are acquired and/or viewed in two orthogonal axes.

3-D
Three-dimensional
Refers to imaging modalities and images in radiology in which data are acquired and/or viewed in three orthogonal axes .

δ
Delta; Δ
1. Used in conjunction with physical quantities to express difference or interval.
2. Shorthand for medical diagnosis.
D, Δx, Dx
(see δδ, ΔΔ, Ddx, Δdx)

δ agent
Delta agent
Virus requiring hepatitis B virus (HBV) for propagation. Causes severe HBV infection in HBV carriers.
HDV, Hep D

d
Day(s)
24 hour period.
6/7

d
Diameter
1. Straight line passing through the centre of a circle, disc or sphere from one side to the other.
2. The length of such a line.

d
Distance between the lead strips of a radiographic grid.
(see D)

d
Object film distance
Distance between a radiographic subject and the film or cassette.
OFD

D
Absorbed dose
Energy absorbed by medium in a small mass.
(see Gy, KERMA)

D
Delta, Δ
See under δ.

D
Diagonal branch
Terminal branch of the left anterior descending coronary artery.

D
Diastole
Cardiac relaxation period.

D
Distance
See under d.

D
Donor
Individual (or animal) from whom a transplanted organ or tissue originates.

D
Dorsal vertebra
Used in conjunction with a number to indicate a particular vertebral level, e.g. D10.
T (thoracic)

D
Duct, ductus
Channel between anatomical structures.

D
Focus–object distance
Distance from the X-ray focal spot to the object being X-rayed.

D
Optical density
Measure of the blackness of radiographic film. $D = \log I_o/I$ (I_o = incident light intensity; I = intensity of light transmitted through film).
OD

D&A
Drugs and allergies
Details of current medication and reactions to previous medications.
(see DH)

D saline
Dextrose saline
Solution of sodium chloride and dextrose for intravenous use.

DA
Developmental age
The age which an individual with a particular level of motor, language and social abilities would be expected to be, based on standardized tables of normal development.

DA

Dopamine
A neurotransmitter. There is an unbalanced deficiency of dopamine in Parkinson's disease.

DA

Drug addict
Individual dependent on narcotic substances.
(*see* IVDA)

DA

Ductus arteriosus
Vessel present in fetal life which connects the main pulmonary artery to the aortic arch; it may persist after birth and cause abnormal shunting.
(*see* PDA)

DAC

Derived air concentration
Annual intake limit for hospital staff of any air-borne radionuclide as stated by the Ionizing Radiation Regulations 1985 (IRR 1985). The annual limit is divided by the volume of air inhaled in a working year.

DA converter

Digital to analogue converter
Electronic component of imaging system which transforms digital data into analogue form.
(*see* AD converter)

DAF

Decay-accelerating factor
Factor present in red cell stroma which protects red cells from complement damage. Deficient in paroxysmal nocturnal haemoglobinuria (PNH).

DAI

Diffuse axonal injury
Shearing CNS injury as a result of severe trauma causing focal white matter lesions.

DAP

Dose area product (meter)
Measure of exposure to ionizing radiation from radiographic equipment.

DAT

Dementia of Alzheimer's type
Commonest acquired cerebral degenerative disease.
AD, ASD

DAT

Digital audio tape
Type of magnetic tape archival medium. Provides high storage capacity and reliability, but deteriorates with time.

dB

Decibel
1. Unit for measuring the intensity of a sound.
2. One tenth of a bel: unit of comparison of the relative power of two (ultrasound) sound beams expressed logarithmically.

dB/dt

Rate of change of magnetic flux density with time. Relates to magnetic resonance imaging.

DBMS

Database management system
Means of organizing large amounts of data on a computer so it can be interrogated very quickly.

DBP

Diastolic blood pressure
Lowest level of systemic arterial blood pressure in the cardiac cycle.
DP

DBS

Double blind study
Investigation in which neither the subjects nor their investigators know which treatment has been assigned to whom. Designed to remove observer bias.

D&C

Dilatation and curettage
Operation to remove the contents of the uterus along with the endometrial lining, often done to investigate (and/or cure) abnormal bleeding.
(*see* ERPC)

DC

Descending colon
The descending part of the left hemicolon.

DC

Direct current
Electric current (i) with net flow of charge in one direction only.
(*see* AC)

DC

Dorsal column
Anatomical neurone column of spinal cord.

DCBE
Double contrast barium enema
Contrast examination of the rectum and
colon, using barium and air as contrast media.
(See Ba, BaFT, BaS, BM)

DCC
Digital compact cassette
Digital recording using a compression code in
'blips' on magnetic tape in a cassette.

DCCV
Direct current cardioversion
Treatment of cardiac arrhythmia using electric
shock applied to the chest wall or directly to
the heart.

DCE
Data communications equipment
A device (like a modem) used to establish and
transfer data across a communications link.

DCG
Dacryocystography
Radiological contrast examination of the tear
duct.

DCIS
Ductal carcinoma in situ
Cancer within breast ducts.

DCM
Dilated cardiomyopathy
Cardiac muscle dysfunction with associated
ventricular dilatation.

DCT
Discrete cosine transform
Type of compression algorithm applied to
digital image data.

DCT
Distal convoluted tubule
Portion of the nephron which fine tunes the
solute balance.

D+d
Focus film distance
Distance between the X-ray focal spot and the
film or film cassette = focus object distance
(D) + object film distance (d).
FFD

δδ
Differential diagnosis
List of possible diagnosis which may explain
particular findings.
ΔΔ, DD, Δdx, Ddx

DD
Developmental delay
Late achievement of normal physical, mental
and social milestones in a child.

DD
Differential diagnosis
See under δδ.
ΔΔ, Δdx, Ddx

DD
Diverticular disease
Herniation of the bowel mucosa through the
muscular layers; thought to be due to increased
luminal pressure produced by colonic muscular
contraction.

DD
Double density
Floppy disk of medium capacity.

DDAVP
1-Deamino-8-D-arginine-vasopressin (desmopressin)
Analogue of antidiuretic hormone used in the
treatment of diabetes insipidus and acute
bleeding from oesophageal varices.

DDC
Diethyldithiocarbamate
Tracer labelled with 201-Thallium used to
study cerebral blood flow (CBF).
(see ^{201}Tl)

DDP
Default display protocol
An arrangement of soft-copy images which
automatically appears on the monitors in a
PACS.

DDU
Duplex Doppler ultrasound
Combination of cross-sectional imaging with
Doppler signal information from a vessel.

Ddx
Differential diagnosis
See under δδ.
ΔΔ, δdx, DD

DDX
Doctor drug exemption
Use of a licensed drug for a non-licensed
application, on a named patient basis.

D=E

Dates equal to examination
Ultrasound assessment of fetal age correlates with age as determined by date of last menstrual period.

DE

Dose equivalent
Product of absorbed radiation dose and a quality factor dependent on the radio-biological effectiveness (RBE) of the radiation.

DEAFF

Detection of early antigen fluorescent foci
Immunofluorescent test specific for cytomegalovirus.

DEFT

Driven equilibrium Fourier transform
Magnetic resonance pulse sequence that uses multiple radiofrequency pulses of varying angles.

desc.

Descending

5% Dex.

5% Dextrose
Solution of dextrose (glucose) isotonic with serum.

Dex.

Dextrose
Simple carbohydrate molecule, central to energy metabolism, and involved in both protein and fat metabolism.
Glu.

DEXA

Dual energy X-ray absorption / absorptometry
Low-dose imaging technique used in bone densitometry and other quantitative tissue measurements.
DXA
(see BMD, HRT)

DF-118

Dihydrocodeine
Opiate analgesic.

DFM

Decreased fetal movements
Less movement than normal detected by mother.

DFP

Diisofluorophosphate
Radionuclide formerly used in white cell labelling.

DFR

Digital fluororadiography
Fluoroscopic images acquired digitally, without film-screen cassettes.

2DFT

2-dimensional Fourier transform
A Fourier transform (FT) mathematical analysis applied along two directions a of a slice of signal data, thereby creating an anatomical image.

3DFT

3-Dimensional Fourier transform
A Fourier transform (FT) mathematical analysis applied along all 3 orthogonal directions of a volume of signal data, thereby creating a high-resolution image in any plane.

DGH

District general hospital
Local hospital providing all basic medical and surgical services. Does not have its own medical school and is not part of a university.

DH

Day hospital
Health care facility offering daytime hospital services to patients resident at home.

DH

Dermatitis herpetiformis
Skin disorder characterized by severe itching and blistering, especially on knees, elbows, scalp and shoulders; associated with coeliac disease.

DH

Drug history
Details of previous and current medication.
(see D&A)

1,25-DHCC

Dehydroxycholecalciferol
Active metabolite of vitamin D.
1,25-(OH)2D3
(see CC)

DHEA

Dehydroepiandrosterone
Major androgen secreted by the adrenal.

DHF

Dengue haemorrhagic fever
Immunologically mediated haemorrhagic disease in patients infected with dengue 2 virus transmitted by mosquito bites, especially in south-east Asia.

DHR
Delayed hypersensitivity reaction
Abnormal immunological response to an antigen occurring more than 12 h after exposure. Associated with viral illnesses and autoimmune disease.

DHS
Dynamic hip screw
Internal fixation device used in the repair of a fractured neck of femur.

DHSS
Department of Health and Social Security
Formerly a UK national departmental body. The department of health (DoH) is now a separate department.

DHT
Di-hydrotestosterone
An androgenic hormone derived from intracellular enzymatic conversion of testosterone in target tissues.

DI
Diabetes insipidus
Failure of water reabsorption in the renal tubules caused by insufficiency of, or insensitivity to, antidiuretic hormone.
(see ADH)

DIB
Difficulty in breathing
Dysp., SOB
(see DOE, SOBOE)

DIC
Direct isotope cystogram
Catheterization of the urinary bladder and injection of radionuclide to assess reflux.

DIC
Disseminated intravascular coagulation
Disorder of diverse aetiology characterized by the consumption of blood coagulation factors in clot formation, leading ultimately to haemorrhage.

DICOM V 3.0
Digital Image Communications in Medicine: Version 3.0.
A detailed specification that describes a standard for formatting and exchanging digital images and associated data for transfer across the interface of an imaging device. Version 3.0 is the latest ACR.NEMA standard.

DIL
Drug-induced lupus erythematosus
Transient lupus syndrome induced by drugs such as procainamide, hydralazine, phenytoin and isoniazid.

DIMSE
DICOM message service element
Command (i.e. service) which is to be carried out according to DICOM protocol specifications.

DIP
Desquamative interstitial pneumonia (US)
Type of interstitial pneumonia with benign course.
(see IPF, UIP)

DIP
Dynamic integral proctography
Investigation of defaecation using rectal contrast medium following electrical stimulation of the anal sphincters.

DIPJ
Distal interphalangeal joint
Synovial joint between the middle and distal phalanges of hand or foot.
TIPJ

DISH
Diffuse idiopathic skeletal hyperostosis
Ossifying diathesis characterized by bone proliferation at the site of tendinous insertions and ligamentous attachments.

DIT
Di-iodotyrosine
Thyroglobulin iodinated with two iodine molecules. These molecules when coupled form thyroxine (T4).
(see MIT, T3)

DJD
Degenerative joint disease
Osteoarthritis.
OA

DKA
Diabetic ketoacidosis
Insulin-deficient state in diabetes causing hyperglycaemia, systemic acidosis and ketonuria.

DKI
Dextrose potassium insulin
Infusion of fluid containing the above, used in the management of glucose homeostasis in diabetic subjects.
GKI

dl
Decilitre
Unit of volume. One tenth of a litre: 10 ml.

DL
Diffusing capacity of the lung
A measure of the ability of oxygen to cross the alveolar membrane and combine with circulating haemoglobin.

DLE
Disseminated lupus erthematosus/discoid lupus erythematosus
Former term for systemic lupus erythematosus (SLE). Now used for discoid lupus erythematosus; a chronic skin disease of unknown aetiology which is probably immunologically mediated.
LE, SLE

DLR
Digital luminescence radiography
Modality using laser read photostimulable phosphor plates (PSP) to produce hard or soft copy digital radiographic images.
CR, DR, PSL

DM
Dermatomyositis
Auto-immune disease affecting skin and muscle.

DM
Diabetes mellitus
Insulin insufficiency or insensitivity resulting in an elevation of blood sugar. Disorder characterized by metabolic abnormalities and long-term damage to eyes, kidneys, nerves and blood vessels.
(see IDDM, MODM, NIDDM)

DM
Diastolic murmur
Turbulent or abnormally directed blood flow, audible on auscultation during the relaxation period of the cardiac cycle.

DM
Doctor of Medicine
Degree awarded by the University of Oxford.

DMA
Direct memory access
Method of sending a whole digital image into main memory without every pixel value passing through the main processor. Allows very fast data transfer. Processor can do other work while the transfer occurs.

DMAD
Dimethylaminodiphosphonate
Tracer labelled with Technetium-99m used for bone imaging.
(see ^{99m}Tc)

DMD
Duchenne muscular dystrophy
X-linked inherited disorder leading to progressive weakness of girdle muscles and eventual respiratory failure.

DMS
Dermatomyositis
Connective tissue disease characterized by progressive symmetrical muscle weakness and calcification with an associated (periocular) heliotrope rash.

DMSA
2,3-Dimercaptosuccinic acid
Tracer labelled with Technetium-99m, used to image the renal cortex.

DMV
Diurnal mood variation
Feature of biological depression.

DN
District nurse
Community-based nurse providing primary health care.

Dn (Dn-1,2,3,4; D-1,2,3,4)
Duodenum (1,2,3,4)
One of the four duodenal segments.

DNA
Deoxyribonucleic acid
Helical molecule made up of deoxyribonucleotides, purines and pyrimidines. Encodes genetic information and forms chromosomes.
(see RNA)

DNA
Did not attend
Used in respect of patients defaulting on their hospital appointments.

DNS
Deviated nasal septum
Deformity or displacement of the nasal septum.

DOA
Dead on arrival
Descriptive term of the state of a patient on arrival at the hospital.
BID

DOB
Date of birth

DOC
Date of conception
Taken as 14 days after the start of the last menstrual period, unless known to be otherwise.

DOC
11-Deoxycorticosterone
An endogenous precursor of corticosterone. Elevated levels occur with biochemical defects in normal steroid synthesis.

DOCA
Deoxycorticosterone acetate
Substance formerly used as mineralocorticoid replacement therapy.

DOE
Dyspnoea on exertion
Shortness of breath when exercising.
SOBOE
(see DIB, SOB)

DOG
deoxyglucose
Metabolic marker which integrates into the glycolytic pathway of cells. Used predominantly in positron emission tomography (PET).
17FDG

DOH
Department of Health
Governmental department responsible for British health care.

DOLV
Double-outlet left ventricle
Aorta and pulmonary artery both arising from the left ventricle.

DOPA
Dihydroxyphenylethylamine
Precursor in the synthesis of adrenaline and noradrenaline from tyrosine. Also a neurotransmitter in the central nervous system (CNS), carotid bodies and sympathetic ganglia.
Dopamine

DOPAMINE
Dihydroxyphenylethylamine
See under DOPA.

DORV
Double outlet right ventricle
Pulmonary artery and aorta both arising from the right ventricle, often with an associated ventricular septal defect.

DP
Diastolic pressure
See under DBP.

DP
Dorsalis pedis (pulse)
Used principally with reference to the palpability of the pulse in one of the arteries supplying the distal foot.

2,3 DPG
2,3-diphosphoglycerate
Endogenously produced substance which increases the oxygen affinity of haemoglobin.

D. Phil.
Doctor of Philosophy
Degree awarded by the University of Oxford.

DPS
Delayed primary suture
Operative technique which involves leaving the wound open initially, with later closure.

DR
Delivery room
Labour suite, where women give birth.

DR
Digital radiography
See under DLR.
CR, PSL

DRC
Diagnostic reporting console
An interactive workstation, with high-resolution monitors for reporting radiological images.

DRESS
Depth-resolved surface spectroscopy
Magnetic resonance spectroscopy technique for obtaining a spectrum at a predetermined depth.

D/S
Dextrose saline
See under D saline.

DS
Double sided
Floppy disk formatted to hold information on both sides.

DS

Disseminated sclerosis
Former term for multiple sclerosis (MS).

DS

Down's syndrome; formerly called mongolism
Trisomy 21 causing a variety of dysmorphic features and a variable degree of mental retardation. Incidence increases with maternal age.

DSA

Digital subtraction angiography
Vascular imaging using computerized subtraction techniques.
(*see IADSA, IVDSA*)

DSH

Deliberate self harm
Self-inflicted injury, e.g. to obtain attention or hospital admission.
SII

DSM (III) R

Diagnostic and Statistical Manual (Third Edition, revised version)
American disease classification manual.

DST

Dexamethasone suppression test
Study of pituitary–adrenal axis, which assesses normal pituitary suppression of adrenocorticotrophic hormone (ACTH) following administration of a potent glucocorticoid. Relevant to the diagnosis of Cushing's syndrome.

DTE

Data terminal equipment
Genetic term for devices that use a computer network.

DTI

Doppler tissue imaging
Doppler ultrasound technique in which tissue movement is displayed in colour while signals from flow are suppressed.
(*see CDI, DTIA, DTIE, DTIV*)

DTIA

Doppler tissue imaging, acceleration
Doppler ultrasound technique in which tissue acceleration is displayed in colour while signals from flow are suppressed.
(*see DTI, DTIE, DTIV*)

DTIE

Doppler tissue imaging, energy
Doppler ultrasound technique in which tissue movement is displayed in colour while signals from flow are suppressed, using energy mode.
(*see CDE, DTI, DTIA, DTIV*)

DTIV

Doppler tissue imaging, velocity
Doppler ultrasound technique in which tissue velocity is displayed in colour while signals from flow are suppressed.
(*see DTI, DTIA, DTIE*)

DTP

Desktop publishing
Software category devoted to producing high quality documents with personal computers.

DTP

Diphtheria, tetanus, pertussis
Combination vaccine given to children in the first year of life to immunize them against the nominated diseases.
(*see MMR*)

DTPA

Diethylene triamine penta-acetic acid
Tracer labelled with Technetium-99m used in renal imaging and the assessment of renal function.
(*see ^{99m}Tc*)

DTs

Delirium tremens
Acute confusional state caused by alcohol withdrawal which is characterized by agitation, visual hallucinations, motor hyperactivity and increased wakefulness.
(*see AOB, C_2H_5OH, EtOH, FAS*)

DU

Duodenal ulcer
Ulceration of the duodenal mucosa.
(*see GDU, GU, HP, H. pylori, PU, PUD*)

D&V

Diarrhoea and vomiting
Passing frequent loose stools and being sick.
(*see GE*)

DV

Deo volentes
Latin for: 'God willing'; if God so wills it.

DV

Ductus venosus
Fetal vein in the liver connecting the
umbilical vein to the inferior cava (IVC) via
the left portal and common hepatic veins.
(see LV)

DVT

**Deep vein thrombosis, deep venous
thrombosis**
Blood clot in deep veins, commonly in
the calf.
(see PE)

DWT

Discrete wave transform
Type of compression algorithm applied to
digital image data.

Dx

Diagnosis
See under δ.

Dx

Disease

DXA

Dual energy X-ray absorption/absorptometry
See under DEXA.
(see BMD, HRT)

DXR

Deep X-radiation
Treatment of neoplastic disease using high
voltage radiation.
DXT, RT

DXT

Deep X-ray therapy
See under DXR.
RT

Dysp.

Shortness of breath.
DIB, SOB
(see DOE, SOBOE)

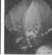

E

e

Base of the natural logarithm
$e = 2.71828...$.

e

Charge of an electron
1.6×10^{-19} Coulomb (C).

e⁻

Electron
Quantum/particle of negative charge
(1.6×10^{-19} Coulomb).

e⁺

Positron
Quantum with the energy of an electron
(1.6×10^{-19} Coulomb) but positively charged.

E

Energy
1. The capacity of a system or radiation to do work.
2. A measure of that capacity expressed in Joules.
(see J)

E

Exposure
Quantity of actinic rays hitting X-ray detector system, e.g. film. The value is proportional to tube current and exposure time.

E/A

Emergency admission
Patient admitted to hospital owing to a critical medical or surgical condition necessitating immediate care.

EAA

Extrinsic allergic alveolitis
Fibrotic lung disease caused by exposure to allergens.

EAC

External auditory canal
Opening of the outer ear.
EAM
(see OE)

EAEC

Entero-adherent E.Coli
Type of Escherichia coli (E. coli) which adheres to bowel epithelium.
(see E.coli, EHEC, EPEC, ETEC)

EAM

External auditory meatus
See under EAC.
(see OE)

EAR

European Association of Radiology
Official European body concerned with the teaching and practice of radiology.
(see ECR)

EBL

Estimated blood loss
Approximate blood loss during a diagnostic, interventional or operative procedure, or after accidental trauma.

eBNF

Electronic British National Formulary
Computerized version of the British National Formulary (BNF) available on compact disk (CD-ROM).

EBT

Electron beam tomography
Extremely fast computed tomography (CT) using a rapidly rotating electron beam and stationary anodes arranged in a circular fashion.
Ultrafast CT

EBV

Epstein–Barr virus
Causative agent of infectious mononucleosis (glandular fever).

EC, E/C

Enteric-coated
Tablet with an outer layer resistant to gastric acid to prevent it dissolving in the stomach.

ECA

External carotid artery
Terminal branch of the common carotid artery supplying areas of the head and neck other than the brain.
(see GF, IM)

ECD

Endocardial cushion defect
Persistence of the primitive atrioventricular canal and anomalies of the atrioventricular valves.
(see CHD)

ECD

Ethylcysteinate dimer
Tracer labelled with technetium-99m for imaging cerebral blood flow.
(*see* ^{99m}Tc)

ECF

Extracellular fluid
Fluid bathing body cells; includes interstitial fluid and intravascular fluid.
(*see ICF, IF*)

ECG (US: EKG)

Electrocardiogram (-graph)
Deflection trace recording of electrical activity in the heart.

Echo.

Echocardiography
Imaging of the heart using ultrasound.
UCG, USCG

ECM

External cardiac massage
Technique for maintaining blood circulation during cardiac arrest.
(*see ABC, AR, BLS, CPR*)

ECMO

Extracorporeal membrane oxygenation
Circulatory bypass of the lungs via external cannulae (usually in right internal jugular vein and left common carotid artery) with artificial oxygenation of the blood outside the body.

E. coli

Escherichia coli
Gram negative bacterium; common gastrointestinal and urinary tract pathogen.
(*see EIEC, VTEC*)

ECR

European Congress of Radiology
Official European radiological meeting.
(*see EAR, ER, RSNA*)

ECS

Endocervical swab
Specimen taken from neck of womb in the investigation of vaginal discharge, looking particularly for gonorrheal infection.

ECT

Electroconvulsive therapy
Electric shock treatment for severe depression.

ECT

Emission computed tomography
Planar method of image acquisition in nuclear medicine, enabling 3-D image reconstruction.
SPECT

EDC

Expected date of confinement
Predicted birth date, i.e. 40 weeks after first day of last menstrual period (LMP). Can be calculated by Naegle's rule: the first day of last menstrual period (LMP) + 1 year – 3 months + 7 days.
EDD

EDD

Estimated date of delivery
See under EDC.

EDE (US:HE)

Effective dose equivalent
Sum of dose equivalents (H) in different body organs multiplied by a weighting factor for each organ (WT). Taking different types of radiation and specific organ sensitivities into account, it gives the effective total body dose.
(*see RBE, Sv, QF*)

EDM

Early diastolic murmur
Turbulent blood flow audible on auscultation early in the ventricular relaxation phase of the cardiac cycle.

EDP

Electronic data processing
Means of manipulating data (often image data) after their acquisition using computer technology.

EDRF

Endothelial derived relaxation factor
Agent secreted by normal blood vessels preventing platelet adhesion.

EDS

Ehlers–Danlos syndrome
Autosomally inherited connective tissue disorder characterized by skin hyperelasticity and joint hypermobility.

EDTA

Ethylenediaminetetraacetic acid
Chelating agent often used as a carrier for radioisotopes. Also used in full blood count (FBC) bottle.

EDV
End-diastolic volume
Volume of blood in the ventricle of the heart just prior to systole (contraction).

EEG
Electroencephalogram
Electrophysiological measurement of activity within the brain.

EF
Ejection fraction
Amount of blood, expressed as percentage of the end-diastolic ventricular volume (EDV), ejected from a ventricle during one cardiac cycle.
(see LVEF, RVEF)

EF
External fixation
Treament of a fracture using pins or other external devices to hold the bone fragments in place.

EFW
Estimated fetal weight
Estimated weight of a fetus in utero.

EG
Eosinophilic granuloma
Granulomatous infiltration of lung and bones; variant of histiocytosis X.

e.g.
exempli gratia (Latin)
For example.

EGA
Extended graphics adaptor
Display card and associated monitor widely used on IBM compatible personal computers.
(see SVGA)

EHEC
Enterohaemorrhagic Escherichia coli
Type of Escherichia coli (E. coli) which adheres to and invades the small bowel epithelium causing a haemorrhagic colitis.
(see EAEC, E. coli, EIEC, EPEC, ETEC, VTEC)

EHL
Effective half-life
Half life for the overall reduction of activity of a radionuclide in the body as a result of both physical and biological processes.
$T_{1/2}eff$

EIEC
Enteroinvasive Escherichia coli
Strains of escherichia coli (E.coli) causing dysentery. They invade colonic mucosa and may cause ulceration.
(see E. coli, EHEC, EPEC, ETEC, VTEC)

EJV
External jugular vein
Main vein draining the scalp and face.
Ext. Jug. V
(see IJV, Int. Jug.V, Jug.V, JV, LIJ, RIJ)

EKG (US)
Elektrokardiogram
See under ECG.

ELF fields
Extremely low frequency fields
1 to 10 mA/m². Currents induced by the application of strong, time varying magnetic fields from clinical magnetic resonance units, or endogenous current densities found in organs such as the brain and heart.

ELISA
Enzyme linked immunosorbent assay
Microscopy technique using specific antibody markers labelled with an enzyme to detect a particular antigenic determinant.The resulting reaction causes a readily visible colour change.
(see IF)

EM
Electron microscope
Instrument for viewing objects too small to be resolved by light beams. Images are formed by electrons from a focused beam which passes through the specimen.
TEM

EM
Erythema multiforme
Non-specific skin disorder characterized by target lesions, often with a central blister, occurring on limbs. Mucosal ulceration may occur. May be precipitated by a number of factors such as viral infections and drugs.

EMG
Electromyograph
Diagnostic test of muscular activity.

E-mail
Electronic mail
System of electronic message transfer between users on the same or linked computer systems, or using modems across telephone networks.

EM pathway

Embden–Meyerhof pathway
Glycolytic pathway in cell metabolism
(anaerobic).

EM radiation

Electromagnetic radiation
Propagation of energy by simultaneous
vibration of electric and magnetic fields,
e.g. X-rays, gamma rays (γ rays). Consisting of
photons, it exhibits both corpuscular and
wave-like properties.
EM wave
(*see EM spectrum*)

EM spectrum

Electromagnetic spectrum
Range of electromagnetic radiation (EM
radiation) including radiowaves, visible light,
micro-, X-, and gamma rays (γ rays).
(*see EM radiation*)

EM wave

Electromagnetic wave
See under EM radiation.
(*see EM spectrum*)

EMD

Electro-mechanical dissociation
Inadequate cardiac output to sustain
apparently normal cardiac electrical activity.
(*see CA*)

EMG

Electromyography
Diagnostic procedure studying the electrical
activity of muscles and nerves.

EMU

Early morning urine
Sample of the first urine voided in the day,
used in pregnancy testing and to look for
mycobacteria when tuberculosis is suspected.

EMU

Energy mode ultrasound
Frequency/directional independent Doppler
technique examining moving objects (blood
cells), with a greater sensitivity than colour
Doppler imaging.

EMW

Early morning waking
Feature of biological depression.

ENA

Extractable nuclear antibodies
Antibodies, found in autoimmune disorders,
(such as scleroderma, Sjögren's,
dermatomyositis), directed against the host's
own nuclear proteins, e.g. scl70.

enc.

Enclosure
Usually typed at the end of a letter to signify
that a further document (or article) has been
included with that transmission.

ENT

Ear, nose and throat
Surgical speciality devoted to the study and
treatment of these organs.

EP

Evoked potential
Neurological test.
(*see VEP*)

EPA

Environmental Protection Agency
US American Federal authority concerned
with radiation protection.

EPA

Erect postero anterior
From back to front, with the subject sitting or
standing. Defines the direction of an X-ray
beam towards a cassette through an erect
subject.

EPEC

Enteropathogenic *Escherichia coli*
Type of *Escherichia coli* which neither adheres
to small bowel epithelium nor produces
diarrhoeaogenic toxins. Its mechanism for
causing diarrhoea is unknown.
(*see E. coli, EIEC, ETEC, VTEC*)

EPI

Echo-planar imaging
Rapid magnetic resonance technique in which
a real-time image is obtained from a slice
selective excitation pulse.

EPISTAR

**Echo-planar imaging with signal targeting
and alternating radio frequency**
Type of echo-planar imaging (EPI) used for
perfusion imaging and magnetic resonance
angiography (MRA).

EPO (Epo)

Erythropoietin
Hormone regulating red blood cell production.
Produced from the combination of a renal
factor with a plasma protein. Also refers to
the synthetic form.
rHuEPO

EPR

Electron paramagnetic resonance
Magnetic resonance phenomenon primarily
involving materials with unpaired electrons.
ESR

EPSI

Echo-planar spectroscopic imaging
Fastest available magnetic resonance
spectroscopy (MR spectroscopy) technique.
(*see EPI*)

ER

European Radiology
Peer-reviewed journal of the European
Congress of Radiology.
(*see ECR*)

ERC

Endoscopic retrograde cholangiography
Contrast study of the biliary system. Involves
endoscopic cannulation of the common bile duct
(CBD) and the injection of contrast medium.
(*see ERCP*)

ERCP

**Endoscopic retrograde
cholangiopancreatography**
Contrast study of the biliary and pancreatic duct
systems performed by endoscopic cannulation.
(*see ERC, ERP*)

ERP

Endoscopic retrograde pancreatography
Contrast study of the pancreatic duct system
involving endoscopic cannulation of the main
pancreatic duct and the injection of contrast
medium.
(*see ERCP*)

ERPC

Evacuation of retained products of conception
Dilatation and curettage to remove the uterine
remnants of an abortion or the placenta post
delivery.
(*see D&C*)

ERPF

Effective renal plasma flow
Value in ml per min of plasma flowing through
kidney.

ERT

Examination room terminal
Computer workstation used to enter and
retrieve patient and exam data from PACS
database during the acquisition of computed
radiography (CR) images.
ET

ERV

Expiratory reserve volume
Maximum volume of air which can still be
exhaled after a quiet expiration.

ESM

Ejection systolic murmur
Turbulent blood flow audible on auscultation,
synchronous with carotid pulsation (i.e.
ventricular systole). Its intensity rises then
falls, being loudest in mid-systole.
SEM

ESN

Educationally subnormal
Mentally retarded individual.

esp.

especially

ESR

Electron spin resonance
See under EPR.

ESR

Erythrocyte sedimentation rate
Velocity of separation of blood cells from
plasma in a test tube. Non-specific marker of
inflammatory or malignant disease.

ESRF

End-stage renal failure
Irreversible loss of kidney function
necessitating dialysis or renal transplantation.
(*see CAPD, CRF, RF*)

ESV

End-systolic volume
Volume of blood remaining in heart ventricle
at the end of a contraction.

ESWL

Extracorporeal shock wave lithotripsy
Treatment for renal or biliary stones by
shattering them using high-energy ultrasound
waves conducted through a bath of water.

ET

Examination terminal
See under ERT.

ET

Endotracheal
Within the trachea. Usually refers to a tube inserted into the trachea to maintain airway patency and /or to facilitate mechanical respiration.
(*see ABC, AR, CPR*)

ET

Endotracheal tube
Tube inserted into the trachea to maintain airway patency and/or facilitate mechanical ventilation.
ETT
(*see ABC, AR, CPR, IMV, IPPV*)

et al.

Et alia
Latin for: 'and other things'. Commonly used for the citation of several authors of a scientific text.

etc.

et cetera
Latin for: 'and the rest', 'and so on'.

ETEC

Enterotoxigenic *Escherichia coli*
Type of *Escherichia coli* which adheres to the small bowel epithelium and produces diarrhoeaogenic toxins.
(*see E. coli, EIEC, EPEC, VTEC*)

EtOH

Ethanol
Ethyl alcohol.
C_2H_5OH
(*see AOB, DTs, FAS*)

ETT

Endotracheal tube
See under ET.

ETT

Exercise tolerance test
Assessment of cardiovascular fitness and potential for cardiac ischaemia using electrocardiographic (ECG) monitoring of a subject on a treadmill or exercise bicycle.
(*see MET*)

EUA

Examination under anaesthesia
(*see MUA*)

eV

Electron volt
Non SI unit of electron energy. Defined as the energy one electron gains when accelerated through one volt potential difference.
$1eV = 1.6 \times 10^{-19}$ J.
(*see e, keV, MeV*)

EVS

Endovaginal sonography (US)
Ultrasound performed by placing the probe in the vagina.
(*see TV*)

Ext.

External
On the outside.

Ext. Jug. V

External jugular vein
See under EJV.
(*see IJV, Int.Jug. V, Jug. V, JV, LIJ, RIJ*)

EZM HD

High density (Barium)
Trade name for high-density barium (250%w/v) used for barium meals.

18F, 18-F
Fluorine-18
Short-lived, beta-emitting radionuclide used in positron emission tomography (PET).
(see β+ emission)

f
Frequency
Repetition rate of a regular event.
Fr., n
(see Hz, λ)

f
Foramen
Hole or canal.
For.

f₀
Larmor frequency
Frequency at which magnetic resonance occurs at a particular field strength for a particular nucleus.
W₀

F
Fahrenheit
Non SI unit of temperature. Formula for conversion to Celsius (C): $1C = \frac{5}{9} \times (F - 32)$.
(see C, K)

F
Faraday
SI unit of capacitance. 1F = 1Coulomb (C) / Volt (V). Named after Michael Faraday (1791–1867).
(see C, SI unit, V)

F
Female

F
Focal spot
Area from which X-rays emanate in tube anode.

F
Focal spot size
Effective size of area from which X-rays emanate in tube anode.

FAP
Familial adenomatous polyposis
Autosomal dominant condition in which multiple polyps occur in the colon. The lesions may become malignant.

FAQ
Frequently asked questions
A compilation of answers to these questions displayed as files by newsgroups on the Internet.

FAS
Fetal alcohol syndrome
Congenital anomalies associated with a high maternal intake of alcohol during pregnancy.
(see AOB, C₂H₅OH, DTs, EtOH)

FAST
Fourier acquired steady state
T2*-weighted rapid gradient echo technique with rewinder gradient to promote steady state. Only applicable to Picker magnetic resonance machines.
GRASS

Fat. Sat.
Fat saturation
Magnetic resonance sequence used to suppress the signal returned from fatty tissues.
(see STIR)

Fax
Facsimile
1. A machine that can scan a page and transmit the image of the page over a telephone line. A receiving machine prints a copy of the original page.
2. The document generated by the fax machine.
3. Now also used as a verb: the act of sending such a communication.
(see E-mail)

FB
Foreign body
Extrinsic material lying within body tissue.

FBC
Full blood count
Quantitative measurements of the major components of blood.
CBC

FBG
Fasting blood glucose
Blood sugar level, measured after a 15 hour fast.

FBM
Fetal breathing movements
Ultrasound assessment of fetal respiration which forms part of a biophysical profile score (BPS).

FD

Film digitizer
Unit which converts conventional film into a digital format, using a laser scanning mechanism.

FD

Floppy disk
Removable plastic computer disk that is low in cost, capacity and speed. Used for information interchange and file backup.

FD

Forceps delivery
Birth *per vaginam* requiring the use of mechanical forceps to extract the baby.

FDA

Food and Drugs Administration
American body for the regulation and licensing of foods, pharmaceuticals, medical devices etc.

FDAW

Film digitizer acquisition workstation
Unit which assimilates the digital image produced by a film digitizer (FD) and sends it to a picture archive and communications system (PACS).

FDDI

Fibre distributed data interface
A network using two fibre optic rings in which the data packets circulate in opposite directions. Operates at a signalling rate of 125 Mbytes/s and a throughput of 12.5 Mbytes/s (approx).

^{17}FDG, 17-FDG

Fluorodeoxyglucose
Metabolic marker which integrates into the glycolytic pathway of cells. Used predominantly in positron emission tomography (PET).
DOG
(*see EM pathway*)

FDP(s)

Fibrin degradation product(s)
Fragments of fibrin breakdown. Elevated blood levels occur in disseminated intravascular coagulation (DIC).

Fe^{2+}

Iron
Metal which is the essential constituent of haemoglobin which binds oxygen (O_2) in red cells.

^{52}Fe, 52-Fe

Iron-52
Short-lived, beta (β)-emitting radionuclide used in positron emission tomography (PET) to image bone marrow.

^{59}Fe, 59-Fe

Iron-59
Isotope used in nuclear medicine for ferrokinetic and *in vitro* red cell studies.

FE

Functional enquiry
Checklist of questions used in medical history taking to ensure no obvious symptoms are overlooked.
ROS, SCL, SE, SR

FEER

Field echo with even echo rephasing
Magnetic resonance (MR) sequence used to demonstrate flowing blood.

Fem.

Femoral
Relating to the femur.

FEV1

Forced expiratory volume in 1 second
Volume of gas exhaled in the first second of forced expiration. A commonly used lung function test.

FF

Filtration fraction
Nephrological parameter.

FF

Fine focus
Type or setting of X-ray tube that produces a narrow radiation beam.

F2F

Face to face
Term used when people who have been corresponding/arguing on the Internet actually meet one another.

FFA

Free fatty acids
Molecules forming triglyceride lipids when esterified to glycol. In blood they circulate bound to albumin providing an important source of energy.
NEFA

FFD

Focus film distance
Distance between the X-ray focal spot and the film or film cassette = focus object distance (D) + object film distance (d).
D+d

FFP

Fresh frozen plasma
Blood product containing human coagulation factors, used intravenously for the acute treatment of bleeding diatheses.

FFR

Fellow of Faculty of Radiologists
Fellowship of this faculty prior to its becoming a Royal college.

FFT

Fast Fourier transform
Fast computational algorithm allowing a periodic function to be expressed as an integral sum over a continuous range of frequencies.

FH

Femoral hernia
Protrusion of mesentery or viscus through the femoral canal.
(see IH)

FH

Family history
Medical or surgical conditions afflicting family members.
FHx

FHC

Familial hypercholesterolaemia
Cause of Friedrickson type IIa hyperlipidaemia. Autosomal dominant defect in binding and internalizing low density lipoprotein (LDL) to its receptor, leading to a markedly increased risk of atheroma.

FHH

Fetal heart heard
Fetal assessment parameter.
(see FHNH)

FHNH

Fetal heart not heard
Fetal assessment parameter. Indication for ultrasound evaluation of fetal well-being.
(see FHH)

FHR

Fetal heart rate
Fetal assessment parameter. Can be measured with ultrasound and forms part of a biophysical profile score (BPS).

FHS

Fetal heart sound

FHx

Family history
See under FH.

FIA

Fistula *in ano*.
Track between perianal skin and lumen of rectum or anal canal.

Fib.

Fibula
One of the two principal leg bones.

FID

Free induction decay
Exponentially decaying electrical signal picked up by surface coils following application of an electromagnetic pulse at resonant frequency in magnetic resonance imaging.
FIS

FIGO classification

A disease classification of the International Federation of Gynecology and Obstetrics
Internationally applied staging system for ovarian cancers.

F_IO_2

Partial pressure of oxygen in inspired air.

FIS

Free induction signal
See under FID.

FISP

Fast imaging with steady state free precession
Pulse sequence in magnetic resonance imaging which uses small flip angles and gradient echoes, but in which phase encoding is reversed after data collection.

FJP

Fell, jumped or pushed
Accident and emergency department (A & E) term for unconscious (or dead) patient found at base of high-rise building. Particularly useful in USA.

FL

Femur length
Assessment of fetal growth using ultrasound to measure the femur during the second trimester of pregnancy.

FLA

Fronto laevo anterior
Position of fetus *in utero*.

FLAIR

Fluid attenuated inversion recovery
Magnetic resonance sequence which suppresses the signal from moving fluid. Used in brain imaging to null the cerebrospinal fluid (CSF) signal.

FLASH

Fast low angle shot
Fast gradient echo magnetic resonance imaging technique that uses gradient reversal alone to form an echo.

FLK

Funny looking kid
Child with dysmorphic features.

FLP

Fronto laevo posterior
Position of fetus *in utero*.

FLT

Fronto laevo transversa
Position of fetus *in utero*.

`Flu

Influenza
Viral infection.

FM

Fetal movements
Assessment of FM forms part of biophysical profile score (BPS) calculated from ultrasound observations.

FMF

Familial Mediterranean fever
Rare inherited disorder of unknown aetiology, characterized by recurrent episodes of fever, peritonitis and pleuritis. Most common in Mediterranean countries. Familial paroxysmal polyserositis

FMP

First menstrual period
Date of onset of menarche.

fn.

Function
1. Purpose, use.
2. Mathematical expression/equation.

FN

False negative
Scientific observation incorrectly deemed to be negative in respect of a particular test. Used in patients with reference to diagnostic tests. Term used in statistics.
(*see* FP, TN, TP)

FNA

Fine needle aspiration
Method of tissue sampling by cellular aspiration through a fine needle, often positioned under imaging control.
FNAB, FNAC

FNAB

Fine needle aspiration biopsy
See under FNA.
FNAC

FNAC

Fine needle aspiration cytology
See under FNA.
FNAB

FNH

Focal nodular hyperplasia
Benign, nodular, well-circumscribed vascular hepatic tumour.

FO

Fronto-occipital
From the forehead to the base of the skull . Defines path of X-ray beam from tube to cassette.

FOB

Faecal occult blood
Traces of blood present in the faeces which can be detected chemically but cannot be seen with the naked eye. May be indicative of gastrointestinal tract disease.

FOB

Fibreoptic bronchoscopy
Investigation of the trachea and bronchial tree by inserting a fibreoptic tube into the large airways.

FOD

Focus to object distance
Distance from the focal spot of an X-ray tube to the object or part being radiographed.

FOI

Fibreoptic interface
A compatible connector linking a modality with a fibreoptic cable.

For.

Foramen
See under f.

FOV

Field of view
(Size of) body area covered by image detector.

FOOSH

Fell on outstretched hand
Description of trauma commonly associated with fractures of the wrist.

FP

False positive
Scientific observation incorrectly deemed to be positive in respect of a particular test. Used in patients with reference to diagnostic tests. Term used in medical statistics.
(*see FN, TN, TP*)

FP

Family planning
Contraception advice services.

FP

Family practitioner
Community-based doctor providing primary health care.
GP

FPDM

Fibrocalculous pancreatic diabetes mellitus
Diabetes mellitus (DM) occurring secondary to chronic pancreatitus..

Fr.

French
Commonly used gauge for catheters and tubes. In radiology most commonly used in respect of angiography catheters.

Fr.

Frequency
See under f.
n
(*see Hz, λ*)

FRC

Functional residual capacity
Resting volume of air in lungs (i.e. at end of tidal expiration).
FRV

FRCP

Fellow of the Royal College of Physicians
Fellowship of the professional body representing physicians in the UK.

FRCR

Fellow of the Royal College of Radiologists
1. Fellowship of the professional body representing radiologists in the UK.
2. The examination usually required to attain Fellowship of the College.

FRCS

Fellow of the Royal College of Surgeons
1. Fellowship of the professional body representing surgeons in the UK.
2. The examination usually required to attain Fellowship of the College.

FRE

Flow related enhancement
Increase in magnetic resonance signal intensity of flowing blood or cerebrospinal fluid relative to stationary tissue owing to the replacement of saturated spins by fully magnetized unsaturated spins.

FRJM

Full range of joint movement
Orthopaedic assessment of mobility denoting normal joint movement.
FROM

FROM

Full range of movement
See under FRJM.

FRS

Fellow of the Royal Society
Member of elite scientific fraternity comprising scientists of international repute.

FRV

Functional residual volume
See under FRC.

F/S

Frozen section
Rapid histological examination of frozen tissue, often performed intraoperatively, dictating surgical resections.

FSD

Focus to skin distance
Distance between the focal spot of an X-ray tube and the skin surface of the subject being irradiated.

FSGS

Focal sclerosing glomerulosclerosis
Renal parenchymal disease causing proteinuria, nephrotic syndrome and renal failure.
(*see CRF, RF*)

FSH

Follicle stimulating hormone
Hormone promoting ovum development prior
to its release from the ovary.

fT4

Free serum thyroxine
Amount of thyroxine in the plasma which is
not bound to protein.

FT

Fallot's tetralogy
Complex congenital cardiovascular
abnormality, comprising a ventricular septal
defect, infundibular pulmonary arterial
stenosis, right ventricular hypertrophy and an
over-riding aorta.
(see BT shunt, CHD)

FT

Fourier transform
A mathematical analysis to decompose a signal
(such as a magnetic resonance signal) into a
sum of cosine or sine waves.
(see FFT)

FT

Full term
Refers to the fetus after 38 weeks gestation.

FTA

Fluorescent treponema antibodies absorbed
Highly specific test for syphilis (Σ) infection.

FTND

Full term normal delivery
Obstetric term for a child born without
complications, after at least 38 weeks
gestation.
FTVD

FTP

File transfer protocol
A system for shifting files across the Internet
(or other network).

FTT

Failure to thrive
Failure to gain weight adequately in infancy.

FTVD

Full term vaginal delivery
See under FTND.

FU, f/u

Follow up
Further information about (or consultation
with) a patient in respect of previous therapy
or observation.

FVC

Forced vital capacity
The total volume of gas exhaled by forced
expiration from full lung volume, a commonly
used lung function test.

FWB

Fully weight bearing
1. Orthopaedic term relating to the patient's
ability to sustain weight in an injured limb.
2. A plaster of Paris cast designed to bear the
full weight of the patient.

FWHM

Full width half maximum
Value for quantifying the linear resolution of
an imaging system in relation to its line spread
function.
(see FWTM, LSF)

FWTM

Full width tenth maximum
Value for quantifying the linear resolution of
an imaging system in relation to its line spread
function.
(see FWHM, LSF)

FYI

For your information

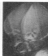

G

γ

Film gamma (γ)

Maximum slope of the approximately linear portion of the characteristic curve of a film. Measure of inherent film contrast.

γ

Gyromagnetic ratio

Ratio of magnetic moment to associated angular moment of the nucleus. Constant for all nuclei of a given isotope. Also called magnetogyric ratio. $\gamma = W_0/B_0$ where W_0 is the Larmor frequency and B_0 the magnetic field.

γ camera

Gamma camera

Standard imaging device in nuclear medicine.

γ decay

Gamma decay

Photon emission from the nucleus of a radionuclide during radioactive decay. γ radiation
(*see* γ *ray*)

γ-GT

Gamma-glutamyltransferase/gamma-glutamyltranspeptidase

Liver and biliary enzyme. An elevated serum level indicates hepatocellular disease and is associated with alcoholism.
GGT

γ-IFN

Alpha interferon(s)

Lymphokines (glycoproteins) released by helper T cells (T_h) with multiple functions, e.g. reducing virus replication and activating macrophages.

γ-LPH

Gamma lipotrophin

Peptide produced from the precursor β-lipotrophin (β-LPH) in melanotrophs of the pituitary pars intermedia.

γ-MSH

Gamma melanocyte stimulating hormone

Peptide produced from the precursor pro-γ-MSH in melanotrophs of the pituitary pars intermedia.
(*see* α-MSH, β-MSH)

γ radiation

Gamma radiation

Photon emission from the nucleus of a radionuclide during radioactive decay (γ decay) or from the anode of an X-ray tube.
(*see* γ *ray*)

γ ray

Gamma ray

Stream of photons emitted during gamma decay (γ decay).
(*see* γ *radiation*)

g

Gram

10^{-3} kilogram (kg).

G

Gauss

Non SI unit of magnetic flux density equal to 1 maxwell/sq. cm. $1\ G = 10^{-4}$ Tesla (T).

G

Gravida

Used with a number to indicate how many pregnancies a woman has had.

67Ga, 67-Ga

Gallium-67

Radionuclide used in the imaging of inflammation, lymphomas and other disorders.

GA

General anaesthetic

General anaesthesia.

GA

Gestational age

Age of fetus *in utero*, usually calculated from last menstrual period.

G&A

Grainger and Allison

Famous textbook of radiology.

GABA

Gamma-aminobutyric acid

Inhibitory neurotransmitter in the central nervous system.

GALT

Galactose-1-phosphate uridyl transferase

Enzyme deficient in the classic form of galactosaemia.

GALT

Gastrointestinal/gut associated lymphoid tissue

Lymphoid tissue within gut wall which can mount an immune response to any antigens encountered.

Gb
Gigabyte
10^9 bytes.

GB
Gall bladder
Sac for storage and concentration of bile prior to its secretion into the duodenum.

GBM
Glomerular basement membrane
Renal membrane between vascular endothelium and glomerulus.
(*see anti-GBM*)

Gbq
Gigabequerel
10^9 Bequerels (Bq).

GBS
Group B Streptococcus
Type of gram-positive bacterium causing neonatal pneumonia.

GBS
Guillain-Barré syndrome
Syndrome characterized by subacute ascending paralysis with areflexia but only mild sensory deficit. There is a marked elevation of the cerebral spinal fluid protein.
AIDP

GC
Gonococcus
Gram-negative bacterium responsible for a sexually transmitted disease (gonorrhoea, 'clap').
Ng

GCS
Glasgow coma scale
System for grading levels of consciousness and neurological dysfunction.

GCSF
Granulocyte colony stimulating factor
Compound used in neutropenic states to accelerate replenishment of the granulocyte (white cell) population.

GCT
Giant cell tumour
Bone tumour (osteoclastoma) which may behave in a benign or malignant fashion.

Gd
Gadolinium
Element used in chelate form as an intravenous contrast medium for magnetic resonance imaging owing to its paramagnetic properties.

GDA
Gastroduodenal artery
Branch of the common hepatic artery supplying stomach, duodenum and pancreas.

Gd-CDTA
Gadolinium cyclohexanediaminetetraacetic acid
Complex (chelate) of an organic ligand and gadolinium which is used as a contrast medium in magnetic resonance imaging.

Gd-DOTA
Gadolinium tetraazacyclododecanetetraacetic acid
Complex (chelate) of an organic ligand and gadolinium which is used as a contrast medium in magnetic resonance imaging.

Gd-DTPA
Gadolinium diethylenetriaminepentaacetic acid
Complex (chelate) of an organic ligand and gadolinium which is used as a contrast medium in magnetic resonance imaging.

Gd-EDTA
Gadolinium diethylenetriaminepentaacetic acid
Complex (chelate) of an organic ligand and gadolinium which is used as a contrast medium in magnetic resonance imaging.

GDU
Gastroduodenal ulcer
Deep focal erosion of the mucosa of stomach or duodenum.
PU, PUD
(*see DU, GU, HP, H. pylori*)

GE
Gastroenteritis
Intestinal infection and/or inflammation causing abdominal pain, nausea, vomiting and diarrhoea.
(*see D & V*)

GE
General Electric
US American electronics company producing imaging equipment.

GE
Gradient echo
Echo produced in magnetic resonance (MR) by reversing the direction of the frequency-encoding magnetic field gradient to cancel out phase shifts.

GET
Gastric emptying time
Time taken for the stomach to empty.
Assessed by scintigraphy of radiolabelled meal.
50% of the radioactivity in the stomach
at time zero should have emptied in
30–60 minutes.

GF
Glandular fever
Common disease of adolescence caused by
Epstein–Barr virus (EBV), also known as
infectious mononucleosis. Its features include
lethargy, lymphadenopathy and splenomegaly.
IM

GFR
Glomerular filtration rate
Renal ultrafiltration rate. Approx. 125 ml/min
per 1.73 m^2 surface area in normal adults.
(*see* CC)

GGT
Gamma-glutamyltransferase/gamma-glutamyltranspeptidase
See under γ-GT.

GH
Growth hormone
Pituitary hormone regulating growth. An
excess causes gigantism in children and
acromegaly in adults.
(*see* GHRH)

GHRH
Growth hormone releasing hormone
A peptide released by the hypothalamus which
stimulates release of growth hormone (GH)
from the anterior pituitary.
GRF

GHz
Gigahertz
Unit of frequency = 10^9 Hz
(cycles per second).

GIF
Graphic interchange format
A format for use in photo-quality images on
the Internet.

GI
Gastrointestinal
Pertaining to the alimentary system (from
month to anus).
(*see* GIT)

GI radiology
Gastrointestinal radiology
Radiology of the GI tract (GIT).

GIFT
Gamete intrafollicular transfer
In vitro fertilization technique whereby ova are
removed, fertilized, and implanted into a
Fallopian tube.

GIH
Gastrointestinal haemorrhage
Bleeding into the gut from the intestinal wall
or from associated organs and appendages
(liver, biliary system, pancreas, diverticula
etc.).

GIS
Gastrointestinal series
Radiological examination of the small and
large bowel, usually with double contrast
barium studies.

GIT
Gastrointestinal tract
The entire alimentary system from mouth to
anus.

GKI
Glucose potassium insulin
Infusion of fluid containing GKI is used in the
management of glucose homeostasis in
diabetics.
DKI

Glu.
Glucose
Simple carbohydrate molecule, central to
energy metabolism, also involved in both
protein and fat metabolism.
Dex.

GM
Grey matter
Macroscopic description of cell nuclei of
central nervous system.
(*see* WM)

GMC
General Medical Council
British body for the registration and regulation
of medical practitioners.

GM counter
Geiger Müller counter
Very sensitive device for detecting and
measuring ionizing radiation.

GM-CSF

Granulocyte macrophage-colony-stimulating factor
Recombinant human growth factor used to reduce the severity of chemotherapy-induced neutropenia.

GMN

Gradient moment nulling
Pulse sequence employed to compensate for flow or motion artifact in magnetic resonance imaging by using gradient magnetic fields to correct for phase errors introduced by motion in a specified direction.

GM plateau

Geiger Müller plateau
Relates to ionization chamber. Occurs at voltage of approx. 900–1200 volt (V) applied between electrodes where the count rate changes only slowly with applied voltage.

GMR

Gradient motion rephasing
Pulse sequence employed to compensate for flow artifacts in magnetic resonance imaging.

GMRH

Germinal matrix related haemorrhage
Intracerebral bleed from vascular tissue adjacent to the lateral ventricles, usually in premature fetuses.

GMRI

Gated magnetic resonance imaging
Magnetic resonance imaging with radiofrequency pulses synchronized with the heartbeat or respiration to avoid motion artefact.

GN

Glomerulonephritis
Immunologically mediated damage to the glomeruli of both kidneys which may be part of a generalized disease.
(see CRF, CGN, RPGN)

GNN

Global network navigator
A browser (i.e. means of sorting information) on the World Wide Web (WWW).

Gn-RH

Gonadotrophin releasing hormone
Hypothalamic hormone regulating the release of gonadotrophic hormones, such as luteinizing hormone (LH) and follicle stimulating hormone (FSH).
(see LHRH)

GOJ

Gastro-oesophageal junction
Anatomical division between stomach and oesophagus.
GOS

GOK

God only knows
Of elusive aetiology.

GOR

Gastro-oesophageal reflux
Abnormal retrograde passage of stomach contents into the oesophagus.
(see GORD)

GORD

Gastro-oesophageal reflux disease
Symptoms and/or signs of disease related to gastro-oesophagal reflux.
(see GOR)

GOS

Gastro-oesophageal sphincter
See under GOJ.

GOT

Glutamatic oxaloacetic transaminase
Enzyme present in liver and heart. Raised serum levels indicate disease of either of these organs.
AST, SGOT

G6P

Glucose-6-phosphatase
Liver enzyme important in glycogenolysis.

GP

General practitioner
Community-based doctor providing primary health care.

G6PD

Glucose-6-phosphate dehydrogenase
Red blood cell enzyme which when deficient (X-linked hereditary disorder) causes an acute haemolytic anaemia in response to an oxidant stress.

GPI

General paralysis of the insane
Dementia and weakness in tertiary syphilis $(3°\Sigma)$.

GPS

Goodpasture's syndrome
Glomerulonephritis caused by antiglomerular basement membrane antibody. Pulmonary haemorrhage may also occur.

GPT

Glutamate pyruvate transaminase
Hepatocellular enzyme. Elevated serum levels
indicate liver disease.
ALT, SGPT

GRAE

Generally regarded as effective
Refers to therapy.

GRAS

Generally regarded as safe
Refers to investigation or, more usually,
therapy.

GRASS

Gradient refocused acquisition in steady state
T2*-weighted rapid gradient echo technique
with rewinder gradient to promote steady
state. Only applicable to General Electric
magnetic resonance machines.
FAST

G&S

Group and save
Determination of a patient's blood group with
retention of a serum sample for subsequent
cross-matching if required.
(see XM, X-match)

GRF

Growth hormone releasing factor
See under GHRH.

GS

Gallstone
Calculus arising in the gallbladder.

GSD

Glycogen storage disease
Autosomal recessively inherited group of
enzyme deficiencies causing abnormal
glycogen metabolism with a variety of clinical
sequelae.

GSS

Gertsmann–Straussler–Scheinker disease
Autosomal dominant disease characterized by
spinocerebellar ataxia with dementia and
plaque-like deposits of amyloid in brain.

G suit

Gravity suit
Compression device used to minimize
haemorrhage in trauma cases.

GSV

Gestational sac volume
Assessment of gestational age, by ultrasound
measurement of intra-uterine gestation sac
during first trimester of pregnancy.

GTN

Glyceryl trinitrate
Vasodilator, predominantly venous, used
intravenously, or sublingually in the
management of angina and heart failure (HF).

GTT

Glucose tolerance test
Investigation to assess disorders of glucose
metabolism by measuring the blood glucose
response to a glucose meal.
OGTT

GU

Gastric ulcer
Ulceration of the gastric mucosa.
(see DU, GDU, HP, H.pylori, PU, PUD)

GU

Genitourinary
Descriptive of the surgical speciality dealing
with lower urinary tract problems and sexually
transmitted diseases (STD).

GUI

Graphical user interface
Methods of interacting with a computer using
a mouse or other pointing device to click on
icons that represent programs, documents or
commands.

GVHD

Graft versus host disease
Rejection by a bone marrow graft of the
patient's own white cells.
G vs HD

G vs HD

Graft versus host disease
See under GVHD.

G$_x$, G$_y$, G$_z$

Symbols for magnetic field gradients; the
subscripts denote the spatial direction of
the gradient.

Gy

Gray
SI unit of absorbed dose (D) of ionizing
radiation. 1 Gy = 1 joule (J)/kilogram (kg).

Gyn.

Gynaecology
Medical speciality concerned with disorders of
the female genital tract.

H₀

Magnetic field
Obsolete symbol for constant applied magnetic field in magnetic resonance.
B₀

H½

Half-value layer
Thickness of an absorber required to reduce X or gamma ray intensity by half.
HVL, HVT
(*see μ*)

H₁

Obsolete symbol for the induced field in magnetic resonance imaging.
B₁

h

Height of lead strips in a grid.

h

Hour
3600 seconds (s).

h

Planck's constant
Ratio of a quantum of radiant energy to the frequency of the associated wave
$h = 6.62 \times 10^{-34}$ J s^{-1}. $h = E/v$ (where E is energy, and v is the wave frequency).

H

Dose equivalent
Product of absorbed dose and quality factor (QF). Takes into account the different radiobiological effectiveness (RBE) of various types of radiation and makes their biological effects comparable.
(*see Sv*)

HA

Haemolytic anaemia
Condition of diverse aetiology characterized by anaemia caused by excessive destruction of red blood cells.

HAM

Human albumin microspheres
Tracer labelled with technetium-99m (^{99m}Tc) used to image lung perfusion in a lung perfusion scan.
V/Q scan

HAPVC

Hemianomalous pulmonary venous connection
Type of partial anomalous pulmonary venous drainage (PAPVD) where one lung drains into the right atrium and the other lung drains normally into the left atrium.
HAPVD, HAPVR
(*see APVR, PAPVC, PAPVR*)

HAPVD

Hemianomalous pulmonary venous drainage
See under HAPVC.
HAPVR
(*see APVR, PAPVC, PAPVD, PAPVR*)

HAPVR

Hemianomalous pulmonary venous return
See under HAPVC.
HAPVD
(*see APVR, PAPVC, PAPVD, PAPVR*)

HAS

Human albumin solution
Protein found in human plasma. Available in commercially prepared form for infusion in hypoalbuminaemic patients.
HSA

HAV

Hepatitis A virus
Liver infection caused by hepatitis A virus.
Hep A

1°HB

First degree heart block
Cardiac conduction defect with delayed electrical conduction between atria and ventricles.

2°HB

Second degree heart block
Cardiac conduction defect with impaired electrical conduction between atria and ventricles, leading to missed ventricular contractions.

3°HB

Third degree heart block
Cardiac conduction defect with complete dissociation between atrial and ventricular activity.

Hb

Haemoglobin
Iron-containing compound found in red blood cells, responsible for oxygen transportation.

HBD

Hydroxybutyrate dehydrogenase
Isoenzyme of lactate dehydrogenase (LD)
found in the heart.
LD

Hb F

Fetal haemoglobin
Molecule found in fetal red blood cells with
high oxygen carrying capacity.
(see Hb)

HBsAg

Hepatitis B surface antigen
Particle detected during acute infection, or the
carrier stage of hepatitis B infection.
HepBsAg

HBV

Hepatitis B virus
Liver infection caused by hepatitis B virus
Hep B

HC

Head circumference
Assessment of fetal development by ultrasound
measurement.

25-HCC

25-Hydroxycholecalciferol
Inactive metabolite of vitamin D precursor to
1,25-dihydroxycholecalciferol (1,25-DHCC).
25-OH-D
(see CC)

HCC

Hepatocellular carcinoma
Primary liver neoplasm.

HCG

Human chorionic gonadotrophin
Hormone produced by a fertilized ovum, which
may be used to confirm pregnancy. Also
produced by malignant germ cell tumours.
β-HCG, B-HCG

HCP

Hereditary coproporphyria
Hepatic porphyria characterized by attacks of
neuropsychiatric dysfunction.

Hct

Haematocrit
Percentage of blood volume composed of red
blood cells.
(see PCV)

HCV

Hepatitis C virus
Liver infection caused by hepatitis C virus
HepC
(see NANB)

HD

Hard disk
Computer storage device consisting of metal
platters sealed inside a case. Stores more data
and accesses them faster than a floppy disc.

HD

High density
Refers to disk storage of high capacity; e.g. a
high density 3½ inch floppy disk holds 1.4 Mb
information.

HD

Haemodialysis
Form of renal replacement therapy where
metabolic waste products are removed directly
from the blood.

HD

Hodgkin's disease
Neoplasm of lymphoid tissue characterized by
Reed–Sternberg cells.
HL

HD

Huntington's disease (chorea)
Inherited (dominant) neurodegenerative
disorder, characterized by late onset disturbances
of movement, mentation and behaviour.

HDL

High density lipoprotein
Lipoprotein important in the transport of
cholesterol from cells.

HDN

Haemolytic disease of the newborn
Fetal anaemia caused by maternal antibodies
crossing the placenta and damaging fetal red
blood cells.
(see Rh)

HDP

Hydrogen diphosphonate
Tracer labelled with technetium-99m (^{99m}Tc);
used in nuclear medicine for bone scanning.
(see EHDP, HMDP, MDP)

HDRBC

Heat damaged red blood cells
Red blood cells altered by heat and labelled
with technetium-99m (^{99m}Tc), used to assess
splenic red cell pooling.

HDU (US: SNF)

High dependency unit
Ward providing intensive nursing care.

HDV

Hepatitis D virus
Virus requiring hepatitis B virus (HBV) for propagation. Causes severe HBV infection in HBV carriers. Also called delta agent.
δ agent, Hep D.

HE

Hypertensive encephalopathy
Rapidly progressive headache, seizures, visual disturbances, altered mental state, and focal neurological signs in patients with uncontrolled elevation of blood pressure.
(*see* BP, HICH, HT)

Helical CT

Helical computed tomography
Form of computed tomography (CT) in which three dimensional (3D) data sets are acquired using a continuously rotating X-ray tube and a moving patient table.
Spiral CT

Hep A

Hepatitis A virus
See under HAV.

Hep B

Hepatitis B
See under HBV.

Hep C

Hepatitis C
See under HCV.
(*see* NANB)

HepBsAg

Hepatitis B surface antigen
Particle detected during acute infection or the carrier stage of hepatitis B infection.
HBsAg
(*see* Hep B)

Hep D

Hepatitis D
See under HDV.

HE stain

Haematoxylin-eosin stain
Common tissue-staining technique used in histology.

Hev

Hepatitis virus
An epidemic water borne hepatitus. A variety of non A, non B hepatitis (NANB).

HF

Haemofiltration
A method of purifying the blood by passing it through a special permeable membrane.

HF

Heart failure
The inability of the heart to maintain sufficient circulation.
CCF, CHF
(*see* LHF, LVF, RVF)

HFD

High fibre diet
Diet containing roughage, i.e. material that passes unabsorbed through the alimentary system.

Hge

Haemorrhage
Bleeding.

HGH

Human growth hormone
Synthetic growth hormone (somatrophin) produced by recombinant genetic engineering; used to treat short stature due to growth hormone deficiency in children.

HH

Hiatus hernia
Protrusion of the stomach through the oesophageal hiatus of the diaphragm.

HHD

Home haemodialysis
Treatment of renal failure by replacement therapy using a blood dialysis machine at home.

HHM

Humoral hypercalcaemia of malignancy
Elevated serum calcium levels as a result of malignant tumours (e.g. lung, breast).

HHT

Hereditary haemorrhagic telangiectasia
Autosomal dominant disorder causing naevi in the skin and gastrointestinal tract which may bleed and arteriovenous malformations of the pulmonary circulation.
OWR
(*see* PAVM)

HI

Head injury

5-HIAA

5-Hydroxindole acetic acid
Breakdown product of serotonin
5-hydroxytryptamine (5-HT). Elevated urinary
levels are present in patients with carcinoid
syndrome.

HIB

Haemophilus influenzae type B
1. Bacterial infection commonly affecting
children in whom it may cause
tracheobronchitis and meningitis.
2. The vaccine against this organism.

HICH

Hypertensive intracerebral haemorrhage
Spontaneous intracerebral bleeding in
hypertensive patients, commonly involving
the basal ganglia, external capsule, and pons.

HIDA

Hepatic iminodiacetic acid
Tracer labelled with technetium-99m (^{99m}Tc)
used to image the biliary system.
IDA

HIE

Hypoxic ischaemic encephalopathy
Perinatal brain injury due to reduced cerebral
blood (and oxygen) supply.

HIG

Human immunoglobulin
Tracer labelled with technetium-99m (^{99m}Tc)
used as a marker for inflammation.

H. influenzae

Haemophilus influenzae
Small, non-spore forming, gram-negative
bacillus (bacterium). A common respiratory
pathogen.

HIPDM

N-trimethyl-n-(2-hydroxyl-3-methyl-5-
iodobenzyl)-1,3-propendiamine
Tracer labelled with iodine-123 (^{123}I) used to
measure cerebral blood flow.

HIS

Hospital information system
Hospital-wide computer network which
manages text data within the hospital.
(*see PACS, RIS*)

Histo(l).

Histology
Microscopic study of tissues.

HIV

Human immunodeficiency virus
Virus causing acquired immunodeficiency
syndrome.
HTLV 1
(*see AIDS*)

H&L

Heart and lungs

HL

Hodgkin's lymphoma
See under HD.

HLA

Human leucocyte antigen
Major histocompatibility gene complex
(MHC) in humans.

HLDLC

High level data link control
An international standard set by the
International Standards Organisation (ISO).
A set of protocols for carrying data over a link
with error and flow control.

HLHS

Hypoplastic left heart syndrome
Congenital heart disease with under-
development of the left ventricle.
HLV
(*see CHD*)

HLTx

Heart–lung transplant
Surgical replacement of diseased heart and
lungs.

HLV

Hypoplastic left ventricle
See under HLHS.

HMD

Hyaline membrane disease
Obsolete term for acute respiratory
insufficiency in premature neonates due to a
lack of surfactant. 'Ground-glass' air-space
consolidation is seen on a chest radiograph.
RDS (current terminology)
(*see ARDS*)

HMDP

Hydroxymethylenediphosphonate
Tracer labelled with technetium-99m (^{99m}Tc)
used in nuclear medicine for bone scanning.
MHDP
(*see EHDP, HDP, MDP*)

hMG

Human menopausal gonadotrophin
Gonadotrophin used for the induction of
ovulation in the treatment of infertility.

HMIBI

Hexakis-2-methoxyisobutylisonitrile
Tracer labelled with technetium-99m (^{99m}Tc)
used in nuclear medicine for imaging the
myocardium and parathyroids.
BIN, MIBI

HMMA

4-Hydroxy-3-methoxymandelic acid
Adrenaline metabolite indicative of
phaeochromocytoma when present in the
urine.
VMA

HMPAO

Hexamethylpropyleneamine oxime
Tracer labelled with technetium-99m (^{99m}Tc)
used to measure cerebral blood flow.

HMSN

Hereditary motor-sensory neuropathy
Autosomal dominant disease involving both
motor and sensory peripheral nerves
characterized by pes cavus, congenital
hip problems and atrophy of the peroneal
muscles.

HNKC

Hyperosmolar nonketotic coma
Metabolic disorder seen in non-insulin
dependent diabetes mellitus (NIDDM).
Characterized by unconsciousness, severe
hyperglycaemia and dehydration without
ketosis.
HONC

h/o

History of
Details of onset and progression of
symptoms which have caused patient to
see a doctor.
HO, H/O, HPC, HPI

HO

History of
See under h/o.
H/O, HPC, HPI

H/O

History of
See under h/o.
HO, HPC, HPI

HO

House officer
Most junior hospital doctor.
PRHO
(*see HP, HS*)

HOA

Hypertrophic osteoarthropathy
Peripheral, symmetrical, bilateral periosteal
reaction affecting wrists and other bones.
Associated with various diseases, classically
lung carcinoma.
HPA, HPOA

HOCM

High osmolar contrast medium
Member of a group of X-ray contrast media
that are characterized by their relatively high
osmolarity.

HOCM

Hypertrophic cardiomyopathy
Cardiac muscle disease characterized by
heterogeneous left ventricular hypertrophy and
ventricular outflow obstruction.

H of F

Height of fundus
Distance of the palpable margin of the uterine
fundus from the symphysis pubis; used to assess
fetal size and growth.

HONC

Hyperosmolar nonketotic coma
See under HNKC.

HONK

Hyperosmolar non-ketosis
Insulin deficient state characterized by
hyperglycaemia, and associated osmotic
diuresis leading to profound dehydration.
Ketoacidosis is absent.

H&P

History and physical examination
Details of a patient's symptoms and of the
clinical findings on examination.

HP

Helicobacter pylori
Bacterium implicated as causal agent in cases
of peptic ulceration.
H. pylori
(*see DU, GDU, GU, PU, PUD*)

HP

Hepatic porphyria
Uroporphyrin decarboxylase deficiency causing light-induced blisters, hyperpigmentation, hirsutism, diabetes and liver neoplasms.
PCT

HP

House physician
Junior doctor on first medical attachment.
(*see HS, SHO*)

HP

Hypersensitivity pneumonitis
Immunologically induced inflammation of the lung, secondary to repeated inhalation of a variety of allergens.

HPA

Hypertrophie pulmonary arthropathy
See under HOA.
HPOA

HPB

Hepatobiliary
Descriptive term including the liver, intra- and extrahepatic bile ducts, gall bladder and pancreas.

HPC

History of presenting complaint; history of present condition
See under h/o.
HO, H/O, HPI

HPD

Home peritoneal dialysis
Treatment of renal failure at home by replacement therapy allowing excretion of metabolic waste across the peritoneum by fluid which is exchanged regularly via a permanent catheter.

HPI

History of presenting illness
See under h/o.
HO, H/O, HPC

HPL

Human placental lactogen
Peptide synthesized by the placenta which is used as a measure of placental function.

HPOA

Hypertrophic pulmonary osteoarthropathy
See under HOA.
HPA

1° HPT

Primary hyperparathyroidism
Elevated level of serum parathyroid hormone (PTH) owing to the presence of one or more secreting parathyroid tumours or parathyroid hyperplasia.
pHPT

2° HPT

Secondary hyperparathyroidism
Elevated levels of serum parathyroid hormone in compensation for a low serum calcium, such as in renal disease.

3° HPT

Tertiary hyperparathyroidism
Elevated level of serum parathyroid hormone owing to autonomous parathyroid hyperplasia. May develop in long-standing secondary hyperparathyroidism.
tHPT

HPT

Hyperparathyroidism
Elevated levels of parathyroid hormone secretion, either primary, secondary or tertiary.

HPV

Hepatic portal vein
Vein formed by splenic and superior mesenteric veins which carries visceral blood to the liver.
PV

HPV

Human papilloma virus
Virus causing warts in humans and associated with various benign and malignant neoplasms.

H. pylori

Helicobacter pylori
See under HP.
(*see DU, GDU, GU, PU, PUD*)

HQ

Headquarters
Centre from which operations are directed.

HRCT

High resolution computed tomography
Technique for computed tomography (CT) using fine cuts and high resolution algorithms, which is especially useful for studying the lung parenchyma.

HRP
High risk pregnancy
Pregnancy at high risk of an abnormal outcome.

HRS
Hepatorenal syndrome
Renal failure secondary to hepatocellular failure characterized by rising urea and creatinine levels with hyponatraemia.

HRT
Hormone replacement therapy
The cyclical administration of oestrogen and progesterone to post-menopausal women and others lacking adequate endogenous production.
(see BMD, DEXA, DXA)

HS
Heart sounds
Sounds emanating from the heart which can be heard with a stethoscope (or the ear alone) during the cardiac cycle.

HS
House surgeon
Junior doctor on first surgical attachment.
(see HP, SHO)

HSA
Human serum albumin
See under HAS.

HSCD
Hand–Schuller–Christian disease
Variant of histiocytosis X characterized by bone defects, pulmonary lesions, exophthalmos and diabetes insipidus.

HSE
Herpes simplex encephalitis
Encephalitis caused by herpes simplex virus.

HSG
Hysterosalpingogram
Injection of contrast medium through the cervical canal, under fluoroscopic screening, to study the uterus and Fallopian tubes.

HSN
Hereditary sensory neuropathy
Autosomal dominant disease characterized by sensory nerve damage resulting in distal mutilation.

HSP
Henoch–Schönlein purpura
A hypersensitivity reaction usually in children after acute infection. Its features include a characteristic rash and painful joints.

HSSD
Hospital sterile supply department
Unit for the storage, sterilization and distribution of sterile dressings, equipment, linen, etc.
HSSU

HSSU
Hospital sterile supply unit
See under HSSD.

HSTAT
Health services technology assessment test
A free electronic resource providing access (via the Internet) to clinical practice guidelines and other full text documents useful for health-care decision making.

HSV
Herpes simplex virus
Deoxyribonucleic acid (DNA) virus causing painful vesicular oral and genital lesions. May persist in a latent form.

HSV
Highly selective vagotomy
Operation for peptic ulcer in which the acid-producing parietal cells are denervated by cutting the terminal vagal nerve fibres.
(see SV)

H&T
Hospitalization and treatment

5-HT
5-Hydroxytryptamine (serotonin)
Biologically active amine produced in the argentaffin cells of the ileum and the appendix. Increased secretion occurs in patients with carcinoid tumours. Also a neurotransmitter.
(see 5-HIAA)

H$_T$
Dose equivalent to individual tissue
Dose equivalent (H) to an individual organ used to calculate the effective dose equivalent (EDE) to the whole body.

HT
Hypertension
Systemic blood pressure raised above 85 mmHg diastolic and 140 mmHg systolic.
(see BP, HE, HICH)

Ht
Height

HTLV 1
Human T-cell leukaemia / lymphotropic virus
Previous name of virus causing acquired immunodeficiency syndrome (AIDS).
HIV

HTML
Hypertext markup language
A set of codes that can be embedded in documents thereby allowing users to interact with linked documents and resources on the Internet.

HTTP
Hypertext transfer protocol
The specification for transmitting multimedia and other information to and from World Wide Web (WWW) servers and client computers on the Internet.

HU
Heat unit
Non SI unit for heat energy produced in X-ray tube.

HU
Hounsfield unit
Measurement of X-ray attenuation used in computed tomography (CT). Numerically compares attenuation of a tissue with that of water.

HUS
Haemolytic uraemic syndrome
Coagulopathy comprising microangiopathic haemolytic anaemia, thrombocytopenia and, commonly, renal impairment.

HVL
Half value layer
See under H½.
HVT
(see μ)

HVS
High vaginal swab
Investigation of vaginal discharge looking for chlamydial (and other) infections. A sample is taken from the external cervical os using a speculum.

HVT
Half value thickness
See under H½.
HVL
(see μ)

HVT
Hepatic vein thrombosis
Clot occluding the veins draining the liver.

HWCD
Hans–Weber–Christian disease
Non-suppurative nodular panniculitis causing skin nodules and multi-system involvement.
WCD

HWP
Hepatic wedge pressure
Method for measuring portal venous pressure by inflating a balloon or wedging a catheter in a hepatic vein.

HWY
Hundred woman years
Statistical term in gynaecology.

Hx
History

HZ
Herpes zoster
Herpes virus causing chicken pox and shingles. Severe infection occurs in the immuno-compromised.
HZV, VZ, VZV

Hz
Hertz
SI unit of frequency.
(see f, kHz, MHz, n)

HZV
Herpes zoster virus
See under HZ.
VZ, VZV

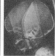

¹²³I, 123-I
Iodine-123
Radionuclide useful for imaging a variety of organs in nuclear medicine. It may be bound to a tracer or used on its own (thyroid imaging).

¹²⁵I, 125-I
Iodine-125
Radionuclide used in nuclear medicine for measuring effective renal plasma flow (ERPF).

¹³¹I, 131-I
Iodine-131
Radionuclide used for imaging the adrenal cortex and the residual tumour and metastases from thyroid cancer. Also used for radiotherapy (RT) of thyroid cancer.

i
Electric current
Flux of electrons.
I
(*see* A)

i
Incisor
Front tooth, for biting (as distinct from chewing).

I
Electric current
See under i.
(*see* A)

I
First cranial nerve (olfactory)
C1, CNI

I
Intensity
Amount of energy (E) of X or gamma rays per unit area and time.

I
Nuclear spin quantum number
Quantifies a property of all nuclei related to the largest measurable component of the nuclear angular momentum.

IA
Intra-arterial
Usually refers to an injection into an artery.

IA
Intra-articular
Within a joint space.

IA
Irradiation area
Area exposed to ionizing radiation.

IAA
Interrupted aortic arch
Developmental obstruction of aorta distal to the left subclavian artery (type A), between the left subclavian and left carotid arteries, or between the innominate and left carotid arteries. The distal blood supply is maintained through a patent ductus arteriosus, which may constrict shortly after birth.
C of A, coarct.
(*see* Ao, CHD)

IABP
Intra-aortic balloon pump
Device inserted into thoracic aorta to increase diastolic aortic pressure and hence coronary and cerebral perfusion. Temporary aid to a failing left ventricle.

IAC
Internal auditory canal
Canal carrying 7th and 8th nerves from the inner ear to the brain.
IAM

IACD
Implantable automatic cardioverter defibrillator
Device used to treat cardiac arrhythmias. A sensor detects ventricular fibrillation and triggers the delivery of an electric shock for cardioversion.

IADSA
Intra-arterial digital subtraction angiography
Arterial imaging from an arterial injection using computerized subtraction techniques.
(*see* DSA, IVDSA)

IAEA
International Atomic Energy Agency
International authority controlling matters related to nuclear energy. Has issued 'Regulations for the Safe Transport of Radioactive Material', guidelines relevant to nuclear medicine.

IAM
Internal auditory meatus
See under IAC.

IAP

Intermittent acute porphyria
Uroporphyrin I synthetase deficiency causing drug and alcohol-induced visceral pain, paralysis, behavioural disturbance and autonomic dysfunction.
AIP

IAS

Interatrial septum
Wall between the left and right atria of the heart.

IBC

Iron binding capacity
Measure of the transferrin (iron binding protein) level in plasma. Elevated in iron deficiency anaemia.
TIBC

IBD

Inflammatory bowel disease
Group of chronic inflammatory disorders of unknown aetiology, including Crohn's disease and ulcerative colitis.

IBI

Intermittent bladder irrigation
Regular flushing of the bladder through an indwelling catheter.

Ibid.

Ibidem
Latin for: "In the same place". Textual annotation when referring to a book, article, chapter or page previously cited.

IBM

International Business Machines
Large firm designing and manufacturing computer hardware and software. 'An IBM' used colloquially refers to their personal computer (PC).

IBS

Irritable bowel syndrome
Syndrome characterized by abdominal pain, distension and flatulence, exacerbated by psychological stress.

IBW

Ideal body weight
Appropriate weight for height.

IC

Inspiratory capacity
Maximum volume of air that can be inhaled from the resting respiratory level, i.e. the end of a normal tidal expiration.
(see FEV, IRC, RV, TLC)

IC

Intracardiac
Within the heart.

IC

Intracerebral
Within the brain.

ICA

Internal carotid artery
Main artery supplying anterior part of brain.

ICA

Islet cell antibodies
Immunoglobulins directed against endocrine cells of the pancreas. More prevelant in some diabetics, their relatives and in pre-diabetics.

ICBG

Idiopathic calcification of the basal ganglia
Calcific deposits in the basal ganglia of the brain. The deposits are of unknown aetiology, and of no clinical significance.

ICD

Implantable cardioverter defibrillator
Implantable device with electrodes passing through the superior vena cava to the right atrium and ventricle which is used to terminate cardiac arrhythmias.

ICD (10)

International Classification of Diseases (10th Edition)
Standard international coding tool for diseases, injuries and related health problems.

ICDS

International Cardiac Doppler Society
Body of cardiac sonographers and sonologists.

ICF

Intracellular fluid
Fluid contained within the body cells.

ICH

Intracerebral haemorrhage
Bleeding into the brain.

ICP

Infantile cerebral palsy
Neurological motor deficit in children caused by hypoxic brain damage at birth.
CP

ICP

Intracranial pressure
Pressure of the cerebrospinal fluid which may be raised in disease and may then produce herniation of vulnerable parts of the brain.

ICR

International Congress of Radiology
Major radiological meeting.

ICRE

International Commission on Radiological Education
International body setting standards in training in radiology.

ICRP

International Commission on Radiation Protection
Advisory body publishing recommendations on dose limitation of ionizing radiation.

ICRU

International Commission on Radiologic Units and Measurements
International body advising on radiological units and measurements.

ICS

Intercostal space
Gap between two ribs.

ICSH

Interstitial cell-stimulating hormone
Anterior pituitary hormone that stimulates ovulation, luteinization and progesterone production in the female, and testosterone production in the male.
LH
(see LHRH)

ICSK

Intracoronary streptokinase
Treatment of cardiac ischaemia by direct injection of the thrombolytic agent streptokinase into the coronary artery.

ICT

Intracranial tumour
Tumour arising within the cranial cavity, i.e. in the brain or its covering membranes.

ICU

Intensive care unit
Ward equipped for acutely ill patients with ventilation facilities and one-to-one nursing care.
ITU
(see RICU)

id

idem
Latin for: 'The same'.

I&D

Incision and drainage
Surgical treatment of an abscess.

ID

Identification
1. Unique characteristics describing person or object.
2. Document describing same.

ID

Infectious disease

ID

Intradermal
Usually refers to injection into the skin.

IDA

Iminodiacetic acid
Tracer labelled with technetium-99m (^{99m}Tc) used to image the biliary system.
HIDA

IDA

Iron deficiency anaemia
An anaemia characterized by red cells that are deficient in haemoglobin (microcytic and hypochromic). The lack of iron may be nutritional or secondary to chronic blood loss.

IDC

Idiopathic dilated cardiomyopathy
Chronic dilatation and dysfunction of the ventricles of the heart, with no obvious cause.

ID card

Identification card
Magnetic card that stores unique information about a patient or system user.

IDDM

Insulin-dependent diabetes mellitus
Form of diabetes mellitus (DM) requiring insulin replacement therapy.
(see NIDDM)

IDE
Integrated drive electronics
A system with simplified electronics for controlling the hard disc. Cheaper than earlier systems, with better reliability and electronic components.

IDL
Intermediate density lipoprotein
Transient intermediary in metabolism between very low density lipoprotein (VLDL) and low density lipoprotein (LDL).

i.e.
id est
Latin for: 'That is'.

IE
Infective endocarditis
Infection of the endothelium lining of the heart commonly in relation to an abnormal or prosthetic heart valve.
BE
(*see* ABE, SBE)

IEC
Intraepithelial carcinoma
Early stage of adenocarcinoma.

IEEE
Institute of Electrical and Electronic Engineers
An organization responsible for many of the standards governing local area networks (LANs).

IEM
Inborn error of metabolism
Congenital metabolic disorder due to an enzyme deficiency or abnormality.

IET
Intrauterine exchange transfusion
Fetal blood transfusion performed *in utero* to treat severe haemolytic anaemia (usually due to Rhesus isoimmunization).

IF
Immunofluorescence
Technique using specific antibody markers that are labelled with fluorescent compounds and examined with a fluorescent microscope.
ELISA

IF
Internal fixation
Treatment of complex fractures using pins placed in bone fragments during a surgical procedure for stabilization of the fracture.
ORIF

IF
Interstitial fluid
Extracellular, extravascular body water compartment.
(*see* ECF, ICF)

IF
Interventional fluoroscopy
Invasive radiological procedures performed under X-ray 'screening'.

IF
Intrinsic factor
Protein produced by gastric parietal cells, essential for the absorption of vitamin B12. Antibodies to the intrinsic factor cause pernicious anaemia (PA).
(*see* RAEB)

IFA
Idiopathic fibrosing alveolitis
Progressive pulmonary fibrosis of unknown cause which predominantly affects lung bases. Causes restrictive defect and low transfer factor.
CFA, FA, UIP

IFA
Immunofluorescence assay
Measurement of antibodies and antigenic material using fluorescein-labelled antibodies.

IFN
Interferon
Substance(s) produced by leucocytes which can now be produced by genetic recombinant techniques and used as antiviral and cytotoxic agents.
(*see* α-IFN, γ-IFN)

Ig
Immunoglobulin
Antibody which can bind antigens (e.g. bacteria) as part of the body's immune defence system.
(*see* IgA, IgD, IgE, IgG, IgM)

IgA
Immunoglobulin A
Antibody found in secretions of the exocrine glands (e.g. tears).
(*see* Ig)

IgD
Immunoglobulin D
Antibody present on surface of many circulating B lymphocytes, and in trace amounts in blood.
(*see* Ig)

IgE
Immunoglobulin E
Antibody mediating acute allergic reactions
(anaphylaxis).
(see Ig)

IgG
Immunoglobulin G
Antibody mediating late response
(within weeks) to bacterial or viral infections.
Part of the body's 'immunological memory'.
(see Ig)

IgM
Immunoglobulin M
Antibody mediating early response
(within days) to bacterial or viral infections.
(see Ig)

IGT
Impaired glucose tolerance
Disorder in which glucose metabolism is
impaired, but to a lesser degree than that
defined by the WHO as constituting frank
diabetes mellitus (DM). IGT exists when the
fasting blood glucose is below 6.7 mmol/l and
the 2hr level following a 75 g oral glucose load
lies betwen 6.7 and 10 mmol/l.

IH
Inguinal hernia
Protrusion of mesentery or viscus through the
inguinal canal.
(see FH)

IHD
Ischaemic heart disease
Reduced heart muscle perfusion, usually due to
atherosclerosis. Causes angina and may result
in infarction.
CHD
(see MI)

IHSS
Idiopathic hypertrophic subaortic stenosis
A presentation of hypertrophic
cardiomyopathy.
(see ASH, HOCM)

II
Image intensifier
X-ray fluoroscopy machine used e.g. for barium
studies, angiography and interventional
radiology.

II
Second cranial nerve (optic)
CII, CNII

III
Third cranial nerve (oculomotor)
CIII, CNIII

IJV
Internal jugular vein
The two internal jugular veins are the
principal draining veins of the brain.
Int. Jug. V
(see Ext. Jug. V, EJV, JV, LIJ, RIJ)

IL-1
Interleukin-1
A factor made by monocytes with various
stimulatory effects on other cells, e.g. it
induces IL-2 synthesis.
(see IL-3)

IL-2
Interleukin-2
A factor (lymphokine) made by T helper cells
(Th) which stimulates proliferation of T cells
and activated B cells.
(see IL-1, IL-3)

IL-3
Interleukin-3
A factor (lymphokine) made by activated
T cells which stimulates all haemopoietic cell
precursors.
(see IL-1, IL-2)

ILF
Idiopathic lung fibrosis
Progressive pulmonary fibrosis of unknown
cause.
CFA, IPF, UIP

ILP
Interstitial laser photocoagulation
The thermal destruction of lesions by laser
energy delivered via percutaneously inserted
optical fibres.

ILV
Independent lung ventilation
Technique to ventilate each lung separately.

IM
Infectious mononucleosis
Common disease of adolescence caused by
Epstein–Barr virus (EBV), also known as
glandular fever. Its features include lethargy,
lymphadenopathy and splenomegaly.
GF

IM
Intramuscular
Usually refers to an injection into muscle.

IMA

Inferior mesenteric artery
The principal artery of the left colon.

IMA

Internal mammary artery
Artery of the anterior thoracic wall, often used in coronary bypass surgery (CABG).
(see LIMA, RIMA)

IMACS

Image archiving and communications system
A hospital-wide network for generating, viewing, archiving and retrieving digital images and their associated reports.
PACS

IMB

Intermenstrual bleeding
Abnormal vaginal bleeding between menstrual periods.

IMHO

In my humble opinion

IMI

Inferior myocardial infarction
Ischaemic death of cardiac tissue resulting from right coronary artery occlusion.
TIMI

IMS

Information management system
The PACS (picture archiving and communications system) database.
(see HIS, IMACS, RIS)

IMP

N-isopropyl-p-iodamphetamine
Tracer labelled with iodine-123 (^{123}I) to measure cerebral blood flow.

IMV

Inferior mesenteric vein
Tributary of the portal vein formed from veins draining the left side of the colon and rectum.

IMV

Intermittent mandatory ventilation
Artificial respiration using regularly delivered breaths.
(see AR, IPPV)

^{111}In, 111-In

Indium-111
Radionuclide used to label white cells for the imaging of possible sites of infection. Also used for labelling platelets.

^{113}In, ^{113m}In

Indium-113m
Radionuclide used in nuclear medicine for blood pool imaging. Forms indium chloride and binds to circulating transferrin.

in.

Inch
Imperial unit of length.
1 inch = 2.7 centimetres (cm).

IN

Interstitial nephritis
Inflammatory cell infiltration of the renal interstitium. May cause acute or chronic renal dysfunction, predominantly affecting the tubules.

inf.

Inferior
Used in anatomical descriptions to denote 'below'.

Ing.

Inguinal
In the region of the inguinal canal, or groin.

Inj.

Injury

INO

Internuclear ophthalmoplegia
Abnormal eye movements associated with a lesion in the medial longitudinal fasciculus. Often due to multiple sclerosis (MS).

INR

International normalized ratio
Laboratory test for monitoring blood clotting especially in patients on warfarin. Ratio of patient's prothrombin time (PT) to a control value.
BCR

Int. Jug. V

Internal jugular vein
See under IJV.
(see EJV, Ext. Jug. V, JV, Jug. V, LIJ, RIJ)

I&O

Intake and output
Record of fluid balance.

I/O

Input / output
The transfer of information into and out of a computer.

IOD

Image object definition
A complete description of the image, according to the DICOM standard, in terms of its attributes (e.g. patient name, image date, etc.).

IOFB

Intra-ocular foreign body
Object or fragment within the globe of the eye.

IOL

Induction of labour
Stimulation of labour by prostaglandin medication or artificial rupture of membranes.
(*see ARM, AROM, ROM, SROM*)

IOP

Intra-ocular pressure
Pressure within the eyeball, normally 15-21 mmHg, elevated in glaucoma.

IORT

Intraoperative radiotherapy
Radiotherapy performed during an operation on a surgically exposed tumour, either directly with a linear accelerator (LINAC) or by the implantation of radioactive seeds.

IOUS

Intraoperative ultrasound
Ultrasound (US) examination performed during an operation on a surgically exposed organ.

i/p

Inpatient
Patient admitted to a hospital or clinic.
IP

IP

Inpatient
See under i/p.

IP

Imaging plate
Photostimulatable phosphor plate (PSP) used to capture a latent radiographic image, later 'read out' by a laser in computed radiographic digital imaging. It is the equivalent of the film-screen combination in conventional radiography.
PPP

IP

Interphalangeal
Joint between two phalanges.
IPJ

IPC

Inter-process communications
Communications between several programs on one or several computers.

IPCD

Infantile polycystic disease
A disorder with autosomal recessive inheritance characterized by small cysts and fibrous tissue in the kidneys and liver.
ARPD

IPD

Intermittant peritoneal dialysis
A limited form of continuous cyclic peritoneal dialysis (CCPD) renal replacement therapy performed for only a few nights each week. Automatic cycler equipment dispenses and drains the dialysis fluid.
(*see APD, CAPD*)

IPF

Interstitial pulmonary fibrosis (US)
Progressive pulmonary fibrosis of unknown cause.
CFA, FA, ILF, UIP
(*see DIP*)

IPH

Idiopathic pulmonary haemosiderosis/haemorrhage
Disorder characterized by recurrent bleeding into the lungs. Bronchoalveolar lavage reveals haemosiderin-laden macrophages.

IPH

Idiopathic pulmonary hypertension
Elevated pulmonary arterial pressure of unknown aetiology.

IPJ

Interphalangeal joint
See under IP.

IPPV

Intermittent positive pressure ventilation
Artificial ventilation whereby gas is intermittently administered under pressure via an endotracheal tube.
(*see AR, IMV*)

IPS

Idiopathic pain syndrome
Pain without a demonstrable organic cause.

IQ
Intelligence quotient
A measure of the intelligence of an individual.
The average IQ = 100 (e.g. cardiologists,
orthopaedic surgeons).

IR
Infrared
Part of the electromagnetic spectrum
comprising waves with a longer wavelength
than those occurring in the visible spectrum.

IR
Interventional radiology
Invasive radiological procedures, usually
therapeutic in nature.

IR
Inversion recovery
Radiofrequency pulse sequence in magnetic
resonance imaging consisting of a 180-degree
pulse followed by a 90-degree detection pulse
to a free induction decay, or a 90-degree and
180-degree pulse pair generating a spin-echo
signal.

IRC
Inspiratory reserve capacity
See under IC.
(see FEV, RV, TLC)

IRR
Ionizing Radiation Regulations
Statute on radiation safety, giving the
maximum permissible limits of radiation
for radiation workers and members of the
public.

IRR 1985
·**The Ionizing Radiation Regulations 1985**
British legal document dealing primarily with
the radiation protection of hospital staff.
ACOP

IRR 1988
**The Ionizing Radiation (Protection of
Persons Undergoing Medical Examinations
or Treatment) Regulations 1988**
British legal document dealing primarily with
the radiation protection of patients.
ACOP

ISBN
International Standard Book Number
Unique number for each book published.

ISDN
Integrated services digital network
National digital (electronic) multi-channel
telephone network providing high speed long
distance links between computer systems.
Suitable for high fidelity transfer of image data.

ISDN
Isosorbide dinitrate
Vasodilator drug used in the treatment of
angina.
ISMN

ISE
Inversion spin-echo pulse sequence
Form of inversion recovery in which a
180-degree inverting pulse is followed by a
90-degree measuring pulse.

ISIS
Image selected *in vivo* spectroscopy
Surface coil gradient method that uses
frequency-selected inversion pulses in the
presence of magnetic field gradients to provide
3D localization of an image volume.

ISIS
International Study of Infarct Survival
Major series of studies into myocardial
ischaemic complications, led by an Oxford
group.

ISO-OSI
**International Standards Organization Open
Systems Interconnection**
A network support protocol for exchanging
DICOM messages.

ISMN
Isosorbide mononitrate
See under ISDN.

ISQ
In status quo
Latin for: 'In the same state'. Used to refer to a
patient's unchanged condition.

IT
Information technology
In hospital setting, refers to speciality
concerned with computerized record of
patients' demographic details and test results,
and its associated supporting hardware and
software.

IT
Injection time
Speed at which an injection, e.g. of contrast
medium, is given.

ITP

Idiopathic thrombocytopenic purpura
Autoimmmune destruction of platelets causing petechial haemorrhage, bruising and, in women, menorrhagia.

ITT

Insulin tolerance test
Test of adrenocorticotrophin (ACTH) reserve by measuring cortisol response to an insulin-induced hypoglycaemia.

ITU

Intensive therapy unit
See under ICU.

i.u.

International Units
Internationally recognized units for assaying biologically active material.
IU

IU

International Units
See i.u.

IU

Intrauterine
Within the uterus.

IUCD

Intrauterine contraceptive device
Copper or plastic implant within the uterus to prevent implantation of the fertilized ovum.
IUD

IUD

Intrauterine death
Fetal death *in utero* after the 23rd week of pregnancy.

IUD

Intrauterine device
See under IUCD.

IUGR

Intrauterine growth retardation
Delayed fetal development.

IUP

Intrauterine pregnancy
Pregnancy that is normally sited within the uterine cavity.

IUT

Intrauterine transfusion
Blood transfusion given to the fetus while still *in utero*.

IV

Fourth cranial nerve (trochlear)
CNIV

IV

Intravenous
Usually refers to an injection into a vein.

IVC

Inferior vena cava
Main vein draining the body below the heart.

IVD

Intervertebral disc
Cartilaginous intervertebral joint.

IVDA

Intravenous drug abuser
Drug addict who uses the venous route for drug administration.
(*see* DA)

IVDSA

Intravenous digital subtraction angiography
Arterial imaging from a venous injection of contrast medium using computerized subtraction techniques.
(*see* DSA, IADSA)

IVF

In vitro fertilization
Extracorporeal technique for fertilizing ova.

IVGTT

Intravenous glucose tolerance test
Measure of response to a glucose load. Demonstrates normality, diabetes or impaired glucose tolerance.

IVH

Intraventricular haemorrhage
Bleeding into the cerebral ventricles.

IVI

Intravenous infusion
Administration of fluid into a vein over a prolonged time period.
(*see* IV)

IVP

Intravenous pyelography
Basic radiographic method for examination of the urinary tract, using an intravenous injection of contrast medium. Intravenous urogram (IVU) is now the preferred term for this procedure.
XU

IVS

Inter-ventricular septum
Wall between the right and left ventricles of heart.

IVU

Intravenous urography
See under IVP. (IVU is now the preferred term for this procedure.)

IVUS

Intravascular ultrasound
Ultrasonographic imaging of vessels (usually arteries) performed by advancing a tiny ultrasound probe within the vessel lumen.

IX

Ninth cranial nerve (glossopharyngeal)
CIX, CNIX

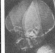

J

Joule
SI unit of work energy.
1 joule is the work done when a force of 1
newton is displaced 1 metre in the direction of
the force. 1 joule (electrical) is the work done
when a current of 1 ampere flows through a
resistance of 1 ohm.

J.

Journal
Jour.

JAMA

Journal of the American Medical Association
Peer-reviewed publication of the American
Medical Association.
J. Am. Med. Assoc.

J. Am. Med. Assoc.

Journal of the American Medical Association
See under JAMA.

JANET

Joint academic network
Network of university and polytechnic
computers linked by the Internet. Originally
based on sites on the Science and Engineering
Research Council (SERC) Network.

JCA

Juvenile chronic arthritis
Spectrum of arthritides in children, Still's
disease accounts for 10%.
(*see JRA*)

JCAT

Journal of Computerized Axial Tomography
Peer-reviewed journal specific to computerized
tomography (CT).

JCD (JKD)

**Jacob–Creutzfeldt disease (Jacob–Kreutzfeld
disease)**
Fatal degenerative disease of the central
nervous system with rapidly evolving dementia
and myoclonus. It is caused by infection with a
slow virus.
CJD, KJD

JD

John Doe; Jane Doe
Initials and names given in US to an
unidentified male or female, respectively.
(*see A.N. Other*)

JE

Japanese encephalitis
Infection with Japanese encephalitis virus,
resulting in fever and headaches, transmitted
by mosquito bites in India, south east Asia,
China and Japan.

JGA

Juxtaglomerular apparatus
Anatomical region of nephron.

JIR

Journal of Interventional Radiology
Official organ of the British Society of
Interventional Radiology.
(*see BSIR*)

JJ

Jaw jerk
Reflex contraction of facial muscles elicited by
tapping the chin.

JJ stent

Double J stent
Internal drainage tube with curves at both
ends. Used in interventional radiology,
especially in urological procedures.

jn.

Junction
Border.

Jour.

Journal
J

JPEG

Joint Photographic Experts Group
Standardization body responsible for a type of
'lossy' compression algorithm applied to image
data.

JRA

Juvenile rheumatoid arthritis
Chronic arthritis in childhood with
rheumatoid factor present in the serum. Mono
or polyarticular synovitis with systemic
symptoms. Still's disease
(*see JCA*)

JSAIR
Japanese Society of Angiography and Interventional Radiology
(see APSVIR, BSIR, CIRSE, CVIR, SCVIR, WAIS)

Jug. V
Jugular vein
Main vein draining the head.
JV
(see EJV, Ext. Jug. V, IJV, Int. Jug V, LIJ, RIJ)

JV
Jugular vein
See under Jug. V.
(see EJV, Ext. Jug. V, IJV, Int. Jug V, LIJ, RIJ)

JVIR
Journal of Vascular and Interventional Radiology
Official organ of the Society of Cardiovascular and Interventional Radiology.
(see SCVIR)

JVP
Jugular venous pressure
Pressure within the internal jugular vein assessed clinically or physiologically, indicating cardiac venous filling pressure.
(see CVP)

JVP
Jugular venous pulse
Triphasic pressure cycle of blood flow in the jugular veins. It reflects right atrial pressure.
(see JVPT)

JVPT
Jugular venous pulse tracing
Recorded waveform of the jugular venous pulse (JVP).

J wire
J wire
Angiographic guide wire with a curved end.

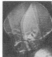

K

k
Constant
Used in equations to describe the relation of physical quantities to each other.

K⁺
Potassium
The principal intracellular ion.

K
Contrast improvement factor
Factor by which grids improve contrast.
K = radiographic contrast (C) with grid / radiographic contrast without grid.

K
Kelvin
SI unit of temperature (T).
(see C, F)

kb
Kilobytes
Literally, 1000 bytes, but in practice 1024 bytes since on the binary system $2^{10} = 1024$, where a byte is a group of 8 bits which can store 256 different values (0–255).

kBq
Kilobequerel
10^3 bequerels (Bq).

KCCT
Kaolin cephalin clotting time
In vitro blood coagulation test.

KCO
Transfer coefficient
Lung function test quantifying the transfer of gas across the alveolar–capillary membrane.

KERMA
Kinetic energy released per unit mass
Kinetic energy (E) of all charged particles liberated by photons in mass (m) of medium.
(see Gy)

keV
Kilo electron volt
1000 electron volts (eV).
(see kV, kVp, MeV)

kg
Kilogram
SI unit of mass. 1 kg = 1000 grams (g).
(see mcg, mg)

kHz
Kilohertz
1000 hertz (Hz).

KJ
Knee jerk
Involuntary contraction of the quadriceps muscle groups in response to passive stretching of its tendon.

KLS
Kidneys, liver, spleen

KO
Knocked out
Rendered unconscious.
Ko'd, KOed
(see LOC)

Ko'd
Knocked out
See under KO.
KOed
(see LOC)

KOed
Knocked out
See under KO.
Ko'd
(see LOC)

kPa
Kilo Pascal
1000 Pascal (PA). Unit of pressure.

Kr
Krypton
Gas used in high-sensitivity ionization chambers for computed tomography (CT).

⁸¹ᵐKr, 81m-Kr
Krypton-81m
Radioactive gas used to assess ventilation in ventilation perfusion (V/Q) scans.

⁸⁵Kr, 85-Kr
Krypton-85
Radionuclide formerly used in nuclear medicine for imaging cerebral blood flow.

KS
Kaposi's sarcoma
Previously rare malignant tumour, usually cutaneous, now commonly encountered in AIDS patients.

KSS

Kearns–Sayre syndrome

Autosomal dominant mitochondrial abnormality, presenting in childhood, characterized by progressive muscular weakness, cardiac conduction defects, retinal pigmentation changes, short stature and gonadal defects.

KTx

Kidney transplant

A kidney that has been transplanted from a donor to a recipient.

Tx kidney

KUB

Kidney ureter bladder

Plain abdominal radiograph to include all of the structures listed.

(see AXR, PAF)

kV

Kilovolt

1000 Volt (V).

(see kVp)

kV

kilovoltage

Potential difference applied between the cathode and anode of an X-ray tube.

(see kVp, V)

kVp

Peak kilovoltage

Peak potential difference applied between the cathode and anode of an X-ray tube. Determines maximum possible energy of emitted photons.

kW

Kilowatt

1000 Watt (W).

KWD

Kimmelsteil–Wilson disease

Diffuse or nodular glomerosclerosis in diabetic nephropathy.

KWS, WKD

(see GN)

KWS

Kimmelsteil–Wilson syndrome

See under KWD.

(see GN)

λ

Lambda
Wavelength.
(see f)

l

Litre
Metric unit of volume. $1\,l = 10^{-3}\,m^3$.
(see ml)

L

Avogadro constant, Avogadro's number
Number of atoms or molecules in one mole
(mol) of a substance.
N, NA

L

Left
(see R)

L

Lumbar nerve root
Used with a number 1–5 to define the root
level.

L

Lumbar vertebra
Used with a number 1–5 to represent a
particular level, e.g. L 3.

LA

Lactic acidosis
Metabolic acidosis caused by the accumulation
of lactic acid in tissues owing to anaerobic
metabolism, secondary to an inadequate supply
of oxygen.

LA

Laser angioplasty
Recanalization of a vascular occlusion by laser
energy to facilitate balloon dilatation
angioplasty.

LA

Left arm
Left upper extremity.

LA

Left atrium
Left heart chamber receiving blood from the
pulmonary circulation.

LA

Local anaesthesia / anaesthetic
1. Numbing of an area of body tissue by the
injection of a pharmacological agent often
derived from cocaine, e.g. lignocaine.
2. (Anaesthetic). The pharmacological agent
producing such anaesthesia.

LAC

Left atrial circumflex
Branch of the main circumflex coronary artery.

LAD

Left anterior descending
Main coronary artery supplying the left
ventricle.
LADA

LAD

Left axis deviation
Abnormal electrical vector of the heart, shown
on an electrocardiogram (ECG).

LADA

Left anterior descending artery
See under LAD.

LAE

Left atrial enlargement
Dilatation or hypertrophy of the left atrium,
usually as a result of outflow obstruction, such
as in mitral stenosis.

LAG

Labiogingival
Pertaining to the lips or gums.

LAG

Lymphangiogram
Contrast imaging of the lymph nodes and
lymphatics.

LAH

Left anterior hemiblock
Type of conduction defect in the heart.
LAHB

LAH

Left atrial hypertrophy
Hypertrophy of the left atrium, usually as a
result of outflow obstruction, such as in mitral
stenosis.

LAHB

Left anterior hemiblock
See under LAH.

LAI

Labioincisal
Refers to an anatomical position between the lips and incisor teeth.

LAM

Left atrial myxoma
Most common benign primary intracardiac tumour. May present with obstruction of the mitral valve or with systemic manifestations.

LAM

Lymphangioleiomyomatosis
Progressive diffuse interstitial lung disease, recurrent chylous pleural effusions and pneumothoraces in premenopausal women.

LAN

Local area network
Interconnected computer systems and terminals on the same or local geographic site.

LAO

Left anterior oblique
Description of a radiographic position in which the left anterior aspect of the patient is nearest to the cassette or film.

lap.

Laparotomy
Exploratory abdominal surgical operation.

Lap.

Laparoscopic
Procedure (e.g. cholecystectomy, appendicectomy) involving minimally invasive surgical instrumentation of the abdomen.

Lap. and dye

Laparoscopy and injection of dye
Laparoscopic visualization of the female pelvic organs, involving transvaginal injection of dye into the uterine cavity to confirm tubal patency.

Lap. steri.

Laparoscopic sterilization
Surgical occlusion of the Fallopian tubes via laparoscope.

LAS

Left anterior superior
Describes an anatomical relationship in which the structure concerned lies in front of and above another reference point.

LAS

Lymphadenopathy syndrome
Prodromal phase of acquired immunodeficiency syndrome (AIDS) with generalized lymphadenopathy.
ARC

Lat.

Lateral
1. Anatomical: lying further from the midline than a reference point.
2. Radiographic: defines orientation of the patient to the cassette, i.e. side on.

Lat. Dol.

Lateri dolenti
With reference to the painful side.

LATS

Long-acting thyroid stimulator
Thyroid stimulating immunoglobulin, probably causes hyperfunction in Graves' disease.

LAV

Lymphadenopathy-associated virus
Previous name of the virus causing acquired immunodeficiency syndrome (AIDS).
HIV, HTLV III

LB

Left bronchus
Main airway to left lung.
LMB
(see RB, RMB)

LBBB

Left bundle branch block
Impaired conduction in the heart causing abnormal interventricular depolarization.

LBP

Low back pain / lumbar back pain

LBW

Low birth weight
Fetus below the third centile for weight at birth.

LCA

Left coronary artery
Main coronary artery supplying the left ventricle and anterior interventricular septum.

LCAT

Lecithin–cholesterol acyltransferase
Enzyme necessary for the esterification of free cholesterol. Deficiency causes premature atherosclerosis.

LCD
Liquid crystal display
Type of lightweight, flat computer screen display.

LCIS
Lobular carcinoma *in situ*
Non-invasive stage of breast carcinoma arising from mammary lobules.

LCM
Left costal margin
Inferior border of the left thoracic cage.

LCx
Left circumflex coronary artery
Branch of left coronary artery supplying the left ventricle.

LD
Lactate dehydrogenase
Enzyme important in lactate metabolism found in the heart, skeletal muscle, liver, kidney, brain and erythrocytes. Its serum level can be a non-specific index of cell damage in these organs.
LDH
(*see HBD*)

LD50
Lethal dose 50
Dose of drug or radiation that would kill 50% of an exposed population. Measure of toxicity.

LD50/30
Lethal dose 50/30
Radiation dose that would kill 50% of an exposed human population within 30 days. Approximately 3–6 Sievert (Sv) for a single-dose total body irradiation.

LDA
Left dorsal anterior
Describes the anatomical position of the dorsum of the fetus relative to the mother.

LDH
Lactate dehydrogenase
See under LD.
(*see HBD*)

LDL
Low density lipoprotein
High molecular weight particle transporting cholesterol to the cells.
(*see IDL, VLDL*)

LE
Lupus erythematosus
Multisystem vasculitis of unknown aetiology, probably immunologically mediated. An important cause of renal disease.
DLE, SLE

LEMS
Lambert–Eaton myasthenic syndrome
Weakness, myalgia and fatigability owing to reduced action of acetylcholine at the neuromuscular junction. Associated with malignancy, especially small-cell carcinoma of the lung.

LES
Lower esophageal sphincter (US)
Physiological sphincter between the distal oesophagus and the stomach.
LOS

LET
Linear energy transfer
Ionizing radiation energy transferred to a medium per unit track length.

LETZ
Loop excision of the transformation zone
Surgical removal of the most distal part of the neck of the uterus for treatment of an abnormal cervical smear (CIN II).

LFD
Large for dates
Fetus larger than expected from the estimated time spent *in utero*. May be the result of maternal disease, such as diabetes.
LGA

LFH
Left femoral hernia
Protrusion of mesentery or viscus into the left femoral canal.

LFT
Liver function tests
Serological levels of bilirubin and liver enzymes used as markers of liver disease.

LFT
Lung function tests
Respiratory function based on spirometric testing.
PRT, RFT

lg.
Common logarithm
Logarithm (log) to the base 10.
log.

LGA

Large for gestational age
See under LFD.

LGD

Limb girdle dystrophy
Inherited disorder causing progressive wasting
of the limb girdle musculature.

LGL

Lown–Ganong–Levine syndrome
Re-entry tachycardia caused by an anomalous
atrioventricular electrical connection (Bundle
of Kent).

LGTI

Lower genital tract infection
Infection affecting the lower urogenital tract,
such as the urethra and vagina. Often sexually
transmitted.

LGV

Lymphogranuloma venereum
Sexually transmitted disease caused by
Chlamydia trachomatis.

LH

Left hand

LH

Luteinizing hormone
Anterior pituitary hormone stimulating
ovulation, luteinization and progesterone
production in the female, and testosterone
production in the male.
ICSH

LHC

Left hypochondrium
Left subcostal region of the abdomen.

LHF

Left heart failure
Inability of the left ventricle to pump blood
adequately. Results in pulmonary congestion
and/or low systemic output.
LVF
(*see CCF, HF, RVF*)

LHL

Left hepatic lobe
Anatomical term used to describe the part of
the liver supplied by the left portal vein and
hepatic artery.
LLL

LHRH

Luteinizing hormone-releasing hormone
Hormone produced by the hypothalamus
which regulates the release of luteinizing
hormone (LH).
(*see FSH, Gn-RH, ICSH*)

LHV

Left hepatic vein
One of the three principal veins draining the
liver into the inferior vena cava.

LHS

Left hand side
On the left.

LI

Lactose intolerance
Lactase deficiency which results in
gastrointestinal symptoms following milk
ingestion.

Li

Lithium
Drug used in bipolar psychiatric disorders, and
resistant depression.

LICA

Left internal carotid artery
Main blood vessel supplying the left side of the
brain.

LID

Large intraluminal density
Density on radiographic studies appearing to
lie within the lumen of a tubular structure.

LIF

Left iliac fossa
Anatomical term referring to the lower left
abdominal cavity below the iliac crest.

LIH

Left inguinal hernia
Hernial protrusion through the left inguinal
canal in the groin. May contain mesentery,
viscera, etc.

LIJ

Left internal jugular
Main vein on the left side of the neck draining
the brain.
(*see EJV, Ext. Jug. V, IJV, Int. Jug. V, JV,
Jug V, RIJ*)

LIMA

Left internal mammary artery
Left anterior chest wall artery often used in
coronary arterial bypass surgery.
(*see IMA, RIMA*)

LINAC

Linear accelerator
Modern radiotherapy machine for high voltage
(V) therapy of tumours.

LIP

Lymphocytic interstitial pneumonitis
Lymphocytic infiltration of pulmonary
interstitium of unknown aetiology with
chronic and progressive course.

LIQ

Lower inner quadrant
Infero-medial quarter, usually of breast.

LJM

Limited joint movement
Indication of possible joint disease.

LJP

Localized juvenile periodontitis
Circumscribed area of infection around a
tooth/teeth in children.

LK

Left kidney

LKKS

Liver, kidney (right), kidney (left), spleen
Abbreviation used when documenting findings
on examination (o/e) of abdominal organs.

L lat.

Left lateral
Left side of patient nearest cassette, film or
image intensifier (II).

LLB

Long leg brace
Type of brace used for supporting a leg which
has been weakened by any cause.

LLC

Long leg cast
Plaster cast used to treat a leg fractured or
injured at a site requiring immobilization.

LLL

Left lobe of liver
See under LHL.
(*see RHL, RLL*)

LLL

Left lower lobe
Posteroinferior anatomical division of the left
lung.
(*see CXR, LUL, RLL, RUL*)

LLLE

Lower lid left eye

LLQ

Left lower quadrant
Non-anatomical term used to describe left
inferior quarter of the abdomen (or breast).

LLR

Large local reaction
Reaction of surrounding tissue to localized
pathology.

LLR

Left lateral rectus
Extra-ocular muscle abducting the left eye.

LLRE

Lower lid right eye

LLZ

Left lower zone
Lower third of the left lung field on a frontal
chest radiograph, below the 4th anterior rib.
(*see CXR, LLL, LMZ, LUZ*)

LMA

Left main artery
One of two main arterial trunks supplying the
heart, arises from the posterior aortic sinus.
LMCA, LMS

LMB

Laurence–Moon–Biedl
Syndrome characterized by retinitis
pigmentosa, polydactyly, mental retardation
and renal anomalies along with obesity,
hypogonadism and, sometimes, diabetes
mellitus (DM).

LMB

Left mainstem bronchus
See under LB.
(*see RB, RMB*)

LMCA

Left main coronary artery
See under LMA.
LMS

LMCA

Left middle cerebral artery
Main terminal branch of the left internal
carotid artery supplying temporal and parietal
cerebral lobes.

LMN

Lower motor nerve/neurone
Motor nerve/neurone directly innervating
muscle.

LMNL
Lower motor nerve lesion
Damage to a motor nerve directly innervating muscle.

LMP
Last menstrual period
Date of onset of last menstruation.

LMR
Left medial rectus
Extra-ocular muscle adducting the left eye.

LMR
Localized magnetic resonance
Technique for obtaining magnetic resonance spectra from regions of interest.

LMS
Left main stem (coronary artery)
See under LMCA.
LMA

LMWH
Low molecular weight heparin
Fractionated heparin which reduces the risk of heparin-induced thrombocytopenia in patients on long-term, low-dose heparin therapy.

LMZ
Left mid zone
Middle third of the left lung field on a frontal chest radiograph, between the 2nd and 4th anterior ribs.
(see CXR, LLZ, LUZ)

ln
Natural logarithm
Logarithm (log) to the base e = 2.71828....
log. e
(see e)

LN
Lymph node
Peripheral lymphoid organs that are connected to the lymphatic circulation by lymphatic vessels.

LNBx
Lymph node biopsy
Sampling of lymphatic tissue for pathological examination.

Lnn
Lymph node(s)
See under LN.

LOC
Loss of consciousness
(see KO, Ko'd, KOed)

LOCM
Low osmolar contrast medium
Member of a group of X-ray contrast media, characterized by their relatively low osmolarity and low toxicity.

log.
Logarithm
The power to which a number, called the base, has to be raised to give another number, usually to the base of 10 (lg).

log. e
Natural logarithm
See under ln.
(see e)

Long.
Longitudinal section
Imaging in a plane along the axial length of a structure.
LS, L/S, Lsect.

LOPP
Chlorambucil, vincristine, procarbazine and premisolene
Chemotherapy regimen.

LOQ
Lower outer quadrant
Infero-lateral quarter, usually of the breast.

LOS (U.S. LES)
Lower oesophageal sphincter
See under LES.

LOSP
Lower oesophageal sphincter pressure
Measurement of the pressure at the lower end of the oesophagus to assess obstruction at this level.

LP
Lumbar puncture
Insertion of a fine needle between two lumbar vertebrae into the sub-arachnoid space to obtain samples of cerebrospinal fluid (CSF).

LPA
Left pulmonary artery
Left division of the main pulmonary artery supplying the left lung.

lp/mm
Line pairs per millimetre
Measure of the spatial frequency (spatial resolution) of a radiographic image. For a conventional chest film it is 5 lp/mm.

LPO

Left posterior oblique
Radiographic position in which the left posterior oblique aspect of the patient lies nearest to the cassette, film or image-intensifier (II).

LPV

Left portal vein
Left branch of the hepatic portal vein.
(*see HPV, MPV, PV*)

LQTS

Long Q–T syndrome
Cardiac arrhythmia diagnosed on electrocardiogram (ECG) by prolonged repolarization which predisposes to ventricular fibrillation.

L–R shunt

Left to right shunt
Pathological connection between the systemic and pulmonary circulations such that blood flows from left heart or aorta back into the right heart or pulmonary artery.

LR

Lateral rectus
Ocular muscle innervated by the sixth cranial nerve. Everts the eye.

LRCP

Licentiate of the Royal College of Physicians
Formerly the basic qualifying degree in (internal) medicine.
(*see MRCS*)

LRD

Living (live) related donor
Individual donating organ/tissue for transplantation into a relative.

LRT

Lower respiratory tract
Pertaining to the airways below the pharynx.
(*see URT*)

LRTI

Lower respiratory tract infection
Infection of the airways below the pharynx.
(*see URTI*)

L/S

Lecithin–sphingomyelin ratio
Assessment of the fetal lung maturity using the ratio of these two substances (protein and lipid) released into amniotic fluid.

LS, L/S

Longitudinal section
See under Long.
Lsect.

LS

Lumbar spine
Vertebral column of the lumbar (lower back) region.

LSC

Left subclavian
Usually in respect of the position of an intravenous line.

LSCS

Lower segment Caesarian section
Abdominal operation to remove an infant from the womb. Standard transperitoneal surgical approach with low transverse fannenstiel incision for Caesarian procedure. Now the commonest type of Caesarian operation.

LSD

Lysergic acid diethylamide
Hallucinogenic 'recreational' drug.

LSE

Left sternal edge
Anatomical term used to describe a location along the left border of the sternum.

Lsect.

Longtudinal section
See under Long.
LS, L/S

LSF

Line spread function
Graph of count rates against distance across a line source of radioactivity. Used in the assessment of spatial resolution.
(*see FWHM, FWTM*)

LSM

Late systolic murmur
Abnormal sound occurring late in the contraction phase of the heart, probably related to papillary muscle dysfunction.

LSR

Liver / spleen ratio
Numerical comparison of the X-ray attenuation values of the liver and spleen as measured by Hounsfield units on a computed tomography (CT) image.

Lt
Left
(see Rt)

LTA
Long-term archive
Archive for long-term digital image storage.
LTS, ODJ

LTM
Long-term memory
Ability to recall events from a long time in the
past.

LTOT
Long-term oxygen therapy (treatment)
Oxygen treatment provided almost
continuously in the home to a respiratory
cripple.

LTS
Long-term storage
See under LTA.
ODJ

LUE
Left upper extremity
Left arm or hand.

LUF
Luteinized unruptured follicle (syndrome)
Condition diagnosed by ultrasound, where a
developing follicle 'traps' the mature ovum,
preventing its release.

LUL
Left upper lobe
Superior anatomical division of the left lung.
(see CXR, LLL, RLL, RUL)

LUO
Left ureteric orifice
Opening of the left ureter into the bladder.

LUOQ
Left upper outer quadrant
Left supero-lateral quarter of the organ under
consideration.

LUQ
Left upper quadrant
Non-anatomical term to describe left superior
quarter of the abdomen (or breast).
ULQ

LUT
Look-up table
A tabulated method of correlating an input
datum value with a related output value, so
that the latter can be easily 'read off' without
any computation being necessary.

LUZ
Left upper zone
Upper third of the left lung field on a frontal
chest radiograph, above the 2nd anterior rib.
(see CXR, LLZ, LMZ, LUL)

LV
Left ventricle
Left heart chamber pumping blood into the
systemic arterial system.
(see RV)

LV
Left ventricular branch
Terminal branch of the right coronary artery.

LV
Ligamentum venosum
Ligament representing the fetal ductus venous.
(see DV)

LVEF
Left ventricular ejection fraction
Amount of blood, expressed as a percentage of
the end-diastolic left ventricular volume,
ejected from the left ventricle during one
cardiac cycle.
EF

LVF
Left ventricular failure
Inability of the left ventricle to pump blood
adequately. Results in pulmonary congestion
and/or low systemic output.
LHF
(see CCF, CHF, HF, RHF)

LVH
Left ventricular hypertrophy
Increased muscular mass of the left cardiac
ventricle of the heart.
(see RVH)

LVOT
Left ventricular outflow tract
Course taken by blood ejected from the left
ventricle past the aortic valve into the aorta.
(see RVOT)

LVWT
Left ventricular wall thickness
Width of the muscle of the left cardiac
ventricle.

M₀

The magnetization vector M₀
Equilibrium value of magnetization directed along the static magnetic field. Proportional to gyromagnetic ratio (g), spin density (N) and static magnetic field (B_0).

μ

Linear attenuation coefficient
Coefficient for X or gamma ray (γ ray) attenuation per unit thickness. Depends on absorber material and beam energy.
(*see H½, HVL, HVT, m/r*)

μF

Microfarad
10^{-6} farad (F). The farad is the derived SI unit of electric capacitance.

μg

Microgram
10^{-6} gm. A metric unit of mass.
mcg
(*see g, kg, mg*)

μGy

Microgray
10^{-6} gray (Gy). The gray is the derived SI unit of absorbed ionizing radiation dose.

μl

microlitre
10^{-6} litre (l).

μs

Microsecond
10^{-6} seconds (s).

μSv

Microsievert
10^{-6} sievert. The sievert is the derived SI unit of dose equivalent.
(*see Sv*)

m

Mass
A physical quantity expressing the amount of matter in a body.
(*see kg*)

m

Metastable
To indicate metastability of a daughter element (e.g. ^{99m}Tc) which, after its creation, undergoes nuclear re-arrangement with emission of gamma radiation (γ radiation).

m

Metre
SI unit of length.
(*see cm, mm*)

m

Molar
Back tooth.

M

Macroscopic magnetization vector
Net magnetic moment of a sample resulting from all the individual microscopic nuclear magnetic moments.

M

Magnification
Factor of magnification of an examined object on an X-ray film or fluoroscopic image.

M

Male

MA

Mental age
Age of a normal individual (usually a child) exhibiting a particular level of mental ability. Used as a reference to assess the degree of mental subnormality based on accepted norms.

MAA

Microaggregates of albumin
Tracer labelled with technetium-99m (^{99m}Tc) used to image lung perfusion in a lung perfusion scan.

Mac

Macintosh
Type of computer made by Apple Macintosh.

MAC

Media access control
Generic term for way in which workstations gain access to transmission media.

MAC

Minimum antibiotic concentration
The minimum concentration of antibiotic causing a 1-log reduction in the number of viable bacteria *in vitro*.
(*see MBC, MIC*)

MAD

Major affective disorder
Psychotic mental illness characterized by
severe mood disturbance.

MAFI

Medic Alert Foundation International
International body which issues 'alert'
bracelets/medallions to individuals with a
serious medical condition, knowledge of which
would alter their medical management in an
emergency situation.

MAG-3

Benzoylmercaptoacetyltriglycerine
Tracer labelled with ^{99m}Tc used in renal
imaging.

MAGIC

**Mucosal and genital inflammation with
inflamed cartilage**
Syndrome which occurs in Behçet's disease.

MAI

Mycobacterium avium intracellulare
Atypical organism causing tuberculosis
especially in immunocompromised patients.

MAL

Mid-axillary line
Imaginary anatomical line extending vertically
downwards from the apex of the axilla.
Effectively the 'midline' of a patient in the
lateral view.

Mammo.

Mammogram
Radiograph of the breast.
Mammography

MAN

Metropolitan area network
Network spanning a geographical area greater
than a local area network (LAN) but less than
a wide area network (WAN).

MAO

Monoamine oxidase
A neurotransmitter.
(*see* MAOI)

MAOI

Monoamine oxidase inhibitor
Class of drugs used as antidepressants; they
prevent the destruction of monoamine
neurotransmitters in the synaptic cleft.
(*see* MAO)

MAP

Mean arterial pressure
The sum of the diastolic blood pressure and
one third of the pulse pressure.

MARC

Machine readable cataloguing
A tagging scheme for bibliographic databases,
used in the production of UK, US (and other)
national bibliographies. Now the standard
exchange format for records.

MARS

**The Medicines (Administration of
Radioactive Substances) Act**
Statutes concerning the protection of patients
or volunteers in clinical research receiving
radioactive substances.

mAs

Milliampere second
Unit of the product of tube current and
exposure time of an X-ray tube.
(*see* A, mA, kV, s)

MAVD

Mixed aortic valve disease
Combination of an incompetent and stenotic
aortic valve, commonly due to rheumatic
fever.

Max.

Maximum
At most, upper limit.

Mb

Megabyte
1 million bytes. Owing to the binary system it
is actually $2^{10} \times 2^{10} = 1,048,576$ bytes.

MBA

Motorbike accident
(*see* MVA, RTA)

MBC

Maximal breathing capacity
The greatest volume of air which can be
breathed by a subject per minute.

MBC

Minimum bactericidal concentration
Lowest level of antibiotic required to kill a
specific bacterium *in vitro*.
(*see* MAC, MIC)

MB. BS

Bachelor of Medicine, Bachelor of Surgery
Primary medical qualification in some
universities (e.g. London).

MB ChB
Bachelor of Medicine, Bachelor of Surgery
(Chirurgie)
Primary medical qualification in some
universities.

Mbq
Megabecquerel
Unit of radioactivity, 10^6 becquerels.
(*see Bq, Ci, Gbq, kBq, mCi, microCi*)

MCA
Middle cerebral artery
Main terminal branch of the internal carotid
artery supplying the temporal and parietal
lobes of the brain.

MC-C
Metacarpo-carpal
Wrist joint between the carpal and metacarpal
bones.

MCDK
Multicystic dysplastic kidney
Failure of normal development of the renal
collecting ducts, tubules and nephrons, with
their subsequent cystic expansion.
MCK

mcg
Microgram
10^{-6} gm.
(*see g, kg, mg*)

MCGN
Minimal change glomerulonephritis
Glomerulonephritis (GN) commonly causing a
nephrotic syndrome (NS).
Minimal change disease.

MCH
Mean corpuscular haemoglobin
Mean red cell haemoglobin.
(*see MCHC*)

MCHC
Mean corpuscular haemoglobin
concentration
Mean red cell haemoglobin concentration.
(*see MCH*)

μCi
Microcurie
10^{-6} curie (Ci). Old unit of radioactivity.
(*see microCi*)

mCi
Millicurie
10^{-3} curie (Ci). Old unit of radioactivity.

MCK
Multicystic kidney
See under MCDK.

MCL
Mid-clavicular line
Imaginary anatomical line extending vertically
downwards from the mid-point of the clavicle
(collar bone).

MCN
Minimal-change nephropathy
Steroid-responsive type of glomerolonephritis
(GN) presenting with nephrotic syndrome
mainly in children.

MCPJ
Metacarpophalangeal joint
Synovial joint between the metacarpal bone
and proximal phalanx.

MCQ
Multiple choice question
Type of examination question presenting the
candidate with a number of possible answers
from which to choose.

MC & S
Microscopy, culture and sensitivity
Standard request for microbiological
examination of a sample or specimen in
suspected infection.

MCTD
Mixed connective tissue disease
Syndrome characterized by a combination of
clinical features similar to those of SLE,
scleroderma, polymyositis, and rheumatoid
arthritis. High serum antibodies to a nuclear
ribonucleoprotein (RNP) antigen are present.

MCU
Micturating cystourethrogram
Contrast examination of the urinary bladder
and urethra obtained by filling the bladder
with contrast medium and imaging during
voiding.
MCUG

MCUG
Micturating cystourethrogram
See under MCU.

MCV
Mean corpuscular/cell volume
Mean red cell volume; haematological index.

MCx
Main circumflex
Major branch of left main-stem coronary artery.

MD
Doctor of Medicine
Postgraduate academic medical qualification in the UK. In the US the degree is the qualifying examination to practise medicine.
(see PhD)

MD
Managing Director

MD
Medical department (US)

MD
Mentally deficient

MD
Mini disc
Digital recording using a compression code in magneto-optically created 'pits' on 2.5 inch plastic disks.

MDIS
Medical diagnostic imaging system
A hospital-wide network for generating, viewing, archiving and retrieving digital images and their associated reports. System used by the American army.
(see HIS, IMACS, PACS, RIS)

MDM
Mid-diastolic murmur
Turbulent cardiac blood flow, audible on auscultation at the mid-point of ventricular relaxation.

MDP
Methylene diphosphonate
Tracer labelled with technetium-99m (^{99m}Tc) used in nuclear medicine for bone scans.
(see EHDP, HDP, HMDP)

MDS
Myelodysplastic syndromes
Acquired bone marrow diseases usually causing anaemia and a low white blood count (WBC). May transform into acute myeloid leukaemia (AML).
(see CML, CMML)

ME
Myalgic encephalomyelitis
Non-specific illness comprising lethargy and lassitude. No significant abnormality identified on investigation. Possible post-viral and/or psychosomatic aetiology.

MEA
Multiple endocrine adenopathy
Syndrome in which two or more endocrine glands harbour functioning adenomas. The condition may be familial and classified according to the organs affected.
MEN
(see MEN (1/2), MEN 1, MEN 2, MEN 2a, MEN 2b, MEN 3)

MEN
Multiple endocrine neoplasia
See under MEA.

MEN (1/2)
Multiple endocrine neoplasia (type 1/2)
Disorder characterized by the development of multiple, benign or malignant tumours of the endocrine system.
(see MEA, MEN, MEN 1 – 3)

MEN 1
Multiple endocrine neoplasia type 1
Disorder comprising tumours or hyperplasia of parathyroids, pituitary and pancreatic islet cells. Does not necessarily always involve all three organs.
Wermer syndrome.
(see MEA, MEN, MEN (1/2) – 3)

MEN 2
Multiple endocrine neoplasia type 2
Disorder comprising parathyroid hyperplasia, phaeochromocytoma and medullary carcinoma of the thyroid. Does not necessarily always involve all three organs.
Sipple syndrome.
MEN 2a
(see MEA, MEN, MEN (1/2) – 3)

MEN 2a
Multiple endocrine neoplasia type 2a
See under MEN 2.
(see MEA, MEN, MEN (1/2) – 3)

MEN 2b
Multiple endocrine neoplasia type 2b
Disorder comprising phaeochromocytoma, medullary carcinoma of the thyroid and mucosal neuromas.
MEN 3
(see MEA, MEN, MEN (1/2) – 3)

MEN 3
Multiple endocrine neoplasia type 3
See under MEN 2b. Mucosal neuroma syndrome.
(see MEA, MEN, MEN (1/2) – 3)

MEP
Message exchange protocol
Defines the rules whereby the sending of
various forms of messages can be set up, carried
out and terminated using the DICOM 3.0
standard protocol.

MET
Maximal exercise text
Limit reached in exercise tolerance test (ETT)
to assess cardiovascular fitness and potential
for cardiac ischaemia during ECG monitoring
of a subject on a treadmill or exercise bicycle.

MET
Modality examination terminal
Workstation used to match up images from a
digital modality with a scheduled exam in the
PACS database.

MeV
Mega electron volt
10^6 electron volt (ev). This order of magnitude
of electron energy is used in radiotherapy.
(see keV)

mF
Millifarad
10^{-3} farad (F). The farad is the derived SI unit
of electric capacitance.

MFH
Malignant fibrous histiocytoma
Malignant soft tissue or bone tumour.

MFV
Maximal flow-volume loop
Relationship between maximal flow rates on
expiration and inspiration.

Mg^{2+}
Magnesium
Chemical symbol for the magnesium cation.

mg
Milligram
10^{-6} gm. A metric unit of mass.
(see g, kg, mcg)

MG
Myaesthenia gravis
Neuromuscular disorder caused by antibodies
against acetylcholine receptors. Characterized
by weakness and easily fatigued skeletal
muscles.

MGUS
**Monoclonal gammopathy of undetermined
significance**
Presence of a homogeneous paraprotein in the
blood on electrophoresis, the importance of
which is unclear.

mGy
Milligray
10^{-3} gray (Gy). The gray is the derived SI unit
of absorbed ionizing radiation dose.

MHC
Major histocompatibility gene complex
Refers to an area of genome coding for proteins
important in self recognition and immune
reactions. The inheritance of these genes plays
a role in the aetiology of autoimmune diseases.
(see HLA)

MHDP
Methylene hydroxydiphosphonate
Tracer labelled with technetium-99m (^{99m}Tc)
used in nuclear medicine for bone scans.
HMDP
(see EHDP, HDP, MDP)

MHV
Middle hepatic vein
One of the three principal veins draining the
liver into the inferior vena cava.

Mhz
Megahertz
Frequency of sound waves used by an
ultrasound probe.
1Mhz = 10^6 cycles per second = 10^6 Hertz.

MI
Mitral incompetence
Cardiac valve disease, in which there is
retrograde flow across the mitral valve back
into the left atrium during systole.
MR
(see MS, MVD, MVS)

MI
Myocardial infarction
Death of cardiac muscle cells due to ischaemia.
(see IHD)

MIB
Management information base
Generic term for database of objects managed
in a network.

MIBG
Meta-iodobenzylguanidine
Tracer labelled with radioactive isotopes of iodine used for the detection of phaeochromocytoma.

MIBI
2-Methoxy 2-methylpropyl isonitrile
Tracer labelled with technetium-99m (^{99m}Tc) used for imaging the myocardium and parathyroids.
(see BIN, HMIBI)

MIC
Minimum inhibitory concentration
Lowest level of antibiotic activity required for anti-bacterial efficacy *in vitro*.
(see MAC, MBC)

micro.
Microbiology
Study of micro-organisms.

microCi
Microcurie
10^{-6} curie (Ci). The curie is an old unit of radioactivity.
(see µCi)

microg.
Microgram
10^{-6} gram (g). The gram is a unit of mass.
(see kg, mcg, mg)

MID
Multi-infarct dementia
Second only to Alzheimer's disease as a cause of progressive, irreversible dementia. Caused by cerebral infarction.
(see AD, ASD, DAT)

min.
Minimum
At least, lower limit.

mins
Minute
60 seconds (s).
(see h)

MIOP
Magnetic iron oxide particles
Magnetic resonance contrast agent which diminishes the signal from normal tissue.

MIP
Maximum intensity projection
Post-processing ray tracing technique for generating three-dimensional (3D) reconstructions in magnetic resonance (MR) and spiral computed tomography (spiral CT), especially angiograms.

MIPS
Millions of instructions per second
Method of rating the raw performance of computers.

MIRD
Medical Internal Radiation Dose Committee
Committee of the Society of Nuclear Medicine dealing with radiation doses in nuclear medicine.

MIT
Mono-iodotyrosine
Thyroglobulin iodinated with one iodine molecule. Coupled with di-iodotyrosine (DIT) it forms tri-iodothyronine (T3).

ml
millilitre
10^{-3} litre (l).

ML
Middle lobe
Central anterior anatomical division of right lung.
RML
(see CXR, RLL, RUL)

MLB
Microlaryngobronchoscopy
Endoscopic examination of the trachea and airways in infants and small children.

MLCN
Multilocular cystic nephroma
Benign neoplasm originating from metanephric blastoma with malignant potential.

MLD
Metachromatic leukodystrophy
Inherited lysosomal disorder, characterized by symmetrical demyelination, and accumulation of lipid material in white matter.

MLF
Medial longitudinal fasciculus
Tract in central nervous system (CNS).

MLSI
Multiple line scan imaging
Sequential line imaging technique that can be used with selective excitation methods in MRI. Adjacent lines are imaged while waiting for relaxation of the first line towards equilibrium. May result in a diminished acquisition time.

mm
Millimetre (US millimeter)
10^{-3} metre (m).

MM
Malignant melanoma
Neoplasm of dermal or retinal pigment cells.

MMA
Middle meningeal artery
Branch of the external carotid artery supplying the dura.

MMAA
Mini-microaggregates of albumin
Tracer labelled with technetium-99m (^{99m}Tc) to image lung perfusion in a lung perfusion scan.

MMFR
Maximal mid-expiratory flow rate
Amount of gas expired during the middle half of a forced expiratory volume curve.

mmHg
Millimetres of mercury
Old unit of pressure still commonly used in medicine. 1 mmHg = 133.322 pascals (Pa).

M-MODE
Motion mode
Ultrasound technique recording the variation of ultrasound amplitude and depth with time. Used in echocardiography.
(*see TM-MODE*)

mmol
Millimole
10^{-3} mole.
(*see mol*)

MMR
Measles, mumps, rubella vaccine
Combined live vaccine given to children during the second year of life.
(*see DTP*)

MMSE
Mini-mental state examination
30 question assessment of patient's cognitive function.
(*see MTS*)

MMVD
Mixed mitral valve disease
The combination of incompetence and stenosis in a mitral valve, commonly due to rheumatic fever.

MND
Motor neurone disease
Neurological disease characterized by progressive muscle weakness, limb and truncal atrophy, and bulbar symptoms and signs.
ALS

^{99}Mo
Molybdenum 99
Radioactive parent of technetium-99m (^{99m}Tc) used in generators.
99-Mo

Mo
Molybdenum
Constituent metal of many X-ray tube anodes, particularly those used for mammography.

MOD
Magnetic optical disc
Device using magnetic and optical technology for erasing and writing data respectively.

MODEM
Modulation demodulator
Device allowing computers to communicate with other computers over analogue telephone lines. Converts digital information to analogue sound and back again.

MODY
Maturity-onset diabetes of the young
Obsolete term for non-insulin dependent diabetes of the young (NIDDY).
(*see IDDM, NIDDM*)

mol.
Mole
SI unit of amount of substance. One mole of a compound has a mass equal to its mass number (A) in grams (g).
(*see mmol*)

MOPP
Mustine, vincristine, procarbazine and prednisolone
Chemotherapy regimen.

MOTSS
Members of the same sex
Gays and lesbians on-line on the Internet.

MPD
Main pancreatic duct
Central draining vessel of the pancreas,
emptying into the duodenum via the ampulla
of Vater.
PD

MPEG
Motion picture experts group
Standardization body responsible for a type of
'lossy' compression algorithm applied to image
data.

MPGR
Multiple planar gradient recalled
Pulse sequence used in fast-scanning
techniques that allow the acquisition of more
than one slice per repetition time.

MPR
Multiplanar reconstruction
Production of 3-dimensional images from
data acquired in a series of 2-dimensional
planes.

MP-RAGE
**Magnetization preparation-rapid acquisition
gradient echo**
Ultra-fast imaging technique.
(see turboFLASH)

MPS
Mucopolysaccharidoses
Storage diseases (types I-VI) due to a
deficiency of lysosomal enzymes, resulting in
organ accumulation of glycosaminoglycans.
(see MPS1, MSSII, MSSIV)

MPS1, MPS1H
Mucopolysaccharidosis 1
Autosomal-recessive deficiency of α-L-
iduronidase, allowing accumulation of
gangliosides. Causes gargoyle-like facies,
dwarfism, kyphosis, hepatosplenomegaly
and severe psychomotor retardation.
Hurler syndrome.

MPS11
X-linked recessive mucopolysaccharidosis.
Hunter syndrome.

MPSIV
Mucopolysaccharidosis with severe skeletal
deformities.

MPV
Main portal vein
Vein formed by the splenic and superior
mesenteric veins which carries visceral blood
to the liver.
HPV, PV

m/r
Mass attenuation coefficient
Coefficient for X or gamma ray (γ ray)
attenuation per unit mass. Depends on
absorber material and beam energy.
(see H½, HVL, m, r)

MR
Magnetic resonance
Imaging technique in which images are formed
by applying a radiofrequency pulse to a subject
in a magnetic field.
MRI, NMR
(see MRS, MRA)

MR
Mitral regurgitation
See under MI.
(see MVD, MVS)

mR
Milliroentgen
10^{-3} roentgen (R). The roentgen is a unit of
dose of electromagnetic radiation.

MRA
Magnetic resonance angiography
Technique for demonstrating vessels and blood
flow using specific magnetic resonance
sequences.
(see MRI)

mrad
Millirad
10^{-3} rad (rd). The rad is a unit of absorbed
ionizing radiation dose.
mrd

MRC
Medical Research Council
Organization responsible for promoting and
funding medical research (UK).

MRCP
**Magnetic resonance
cholangiopancreatography**
Three dimensional (3D) imaging of the biliary
system and pancreatic duct with magnetic
resonance (MR).
(see ERCP)

MRCP
Member of the Royal College of Physicians
1. Membership of the professional body
representing internal medicine in London.
2. The membership examination of the Royal
College of Physicians which, with due
accreditation, grants the status of a specialist
in (internal) medicine.

MRCS
Member of the Royal College of Surgeons
Formerly the qualifying basic medical degree in
surgery.
(see LRCP)

mrd
Millirad
See under mrad.

MRI
Magnetic resonance imaging
See under MR.
NMR

MRI scan
Magnetic resonance imaging scan
1. Image or set of images obtained with a
magnetic resonance imaging scanner
(MRI scanner).
2. The procedure whereby such images are
acquired.
(see MRI)

MRI scanner
Magnetic resonance imaging scanner
Magnetic resonance imaging (MRI) machine.

MRM
Magnetic resonance mammography
Breast imaging using magnetic resonance
imaging (MRI).

mRNA
Messenger ribonucleic acid
Nucleic acid used in copying deoxyribonucleic
acid (DNA) for cell replication.
(see RNA)

MRS
Magnetic resonance spectroscopy
Use of magnetic resonance to obtain spectral
information from specific chemical entities in
compounds or tissues in the form of peaks
analysed according to their frequency,
amplitude and area under the peak.
(see MRA, MRI)

MRSA
**Methicillin-resistant *Staphylococcus
aureus* / Multi-resistant
*Staphylococcus aureus***
Penicillinase-resistant bacterium, against
which β-lactam antibiotics are ineffective.

MS
Mitral stenosis
Narrowing of the mitral valve aperture,
commonly by rheumatic fever.
MVS

MS
Multiple sclerosis
Demyelinating disease, probably
immunological in nature characterized by the
presence of disseminated demyelinated plaques
throughout the central nervous system (CNS).
Commonly follows a progressive relapsing and
remitting course of neurological dysfunction.
DS

ms
Millisecond
10^{-3} seconds (s).

MSc
Master of Science
Postgraduate academic qualification.

MS-DOS
Microsoft disc operating system
The version of the DOS program sold and
supported directly by Microsoft.

MSE
Mental state examination
Assessment of potential psychiatric symptoms
and higher cerebral function.

MSH
Melanocyte stimulating hormone
Pituitary hormone stimulating pigment
production in melanocytes. Raised levels are
associated with Cushing's and Nelson's
syndromes.

MSU
Midstream urine
Clean sample of urine obtained during
voiding.

mSv
Millisievert
10^{-3} sievert. The sievert is the derived SI unit
of dose equivalent.
(see Sv)

MT
Magnetization transfer
Magnetic resonance imaging (MRI) technique based on cross relaxation between 'bound' and 'free' bulk water protons. Provides high lesion–white matter contrast in brain imaging.

MTBF
Mean time between failure
Term used by manufacturers to describe reliability of equipment.

MTC
Medullary thyroid carcinoma
Thyroid malignancy, may be part of a multiple endocrine neoplastic syndrome.
(see MEA, MEN)

MTF
Modulation transfer function
Mathematical tool for quantifying the resolution of an imaging system in relation to spatial frequencies.

MTPJ
Metatarsophalangeal joint
Synovial joint between a metatarsal bone and its related proximal phalanx.

MTR
Magnetization transfer ratio
Ratio quantifying magnetization transfer (MT). $MTR = (M_0 - M_S) / M_0$, where M_0 = tissue signal before MT pulse, M_S = tissue signal when MT pulse is switched on.
(see MRI)

MTX
Methotrexate
A folic acid analogue which blocks its metabolism. Mainly a chemotherapy drug to treat certain malignancies.

MU
Motion unsharpness
Caused by motion of the examined object (patient) during exposure. Patient unsharpness.
U

MUA
Manipulation under anaesthesia
Specialized movements, usually of joints or fractures, performed under anaesthesia.
(see EUA)

MUGA
Multi-gated acquisitions
Method used in nuclear medicine for imaging the heart in relation to the cardiac cycle.

MUMPS
Massachusetts general utility multi-programming system
A computer language useful for minicomputer hardware in dedicated application environments.

MV
Mitral valve
Heart valve lying between the left atrium and left ventricle.

MVA
Motor vehicle accident (US)
RTA
(see MBA)

MVD
Mitral valve disease
Disordered performance of the cardiac mitral valve, which may have a variety of causes.

MVR
Mitral valve replacement/repair
Replacement or repair of diseased mitral valve.

MVS
Mitral valve stenosis
See under MS.
(see MI, MR, MVD)

MW
Mallory–Weiss tear
Longitudinal mucosal split in the oesophagus which often occurs after prolonged retching or vomiting.

Mx
Mastectomy
Removal of the breast in the treatment of carcinoma.

Mx.y
Transverse magnetization
Components of macroscopic magnetization vector at right angles to the static magnetic field in magnetic resonance imaging (MRI).

Mz
Longitudinal magnetization
Component of the macroscopic magnetization along the static magnetic field in magnetic resonance imaging (MRI). It will approach equilibrium (M_o) following excitation by a radiofrequency pulse.

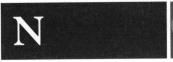
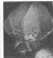

N₂
Nitrogen
Gaseous state of nitrogen (N).
N

¹³N, 13-N
Nitrogen-13
Short-lived beta-emitting radionuclide used in positron emission tomography (PET).
(*see β⁺ emission*)

n
Frequency
Repetition rate of a regular event.
f
(*see Hz, λ*)

n
Number
Quantity of units or events, usually the same or similar in nature.

N
Avogadro constant, Avogadro's number
Number of atoms or molecules in one mole (mol) of a substance.
L, NA

N
Nausea
Feeling sick.

N
Nitrogen
Chemical element forming nearly 80% of the earth's atmosphere.
N₂

N
Signal size
Strength of a signal (commonly number of photons) recorded per pixel by an imaging system.

N saline
Normal saline
0.9% solution of sodium chloride, isotonic with plasma; used in intravenous fluid replacement.
NS

NA
Avogadro constant, Avogadro's number
See under N.

NA
Noradrenaline (US: norepinephrine)
Catecholamine produced at the sympathetic nerve endings. Synthetic precursor of adrenaline.
(*see ADR, DOPA, DOPamine, NADR*)

Na⁺
Sodium
The chief extracellular ion.

NAC
N-acetyl cysteine
Drug used in the acute management of paracetamol poisoning.

Nacq
Number of acquisitions
Number of times an individual slice or volume is sampled in magnetic resonance imaging (MRI), typically 2–4. The higher the Nacq, the better the signal-to-noise ratio (SNR).

NAD
Nicotinamide adenine dinucleotide
Co-factor in oxidation–reduction reactions. Deficient in pellagra.
NADP

NAD
Nothing abnormal detected /Not actually done!
Abbreviation commonly used in clinical notes.
WNL

NADP
Nicotinamide adenine dinucleotide phosphate
See under NAD.

NADR
Noradrenaline (US: norepinephrine)
See under NA.
(*see ADR, DOPA, DOPamine,*)

NAI
Non-accidental injury
Deliberate harm, usually to a child.

NaI(Tl)
Sodium iodide crystal with 0.1% thallium
Scintillator crystal used for imaging in a gamma camera and scintillation detector.

NANB

Hepatitis non-A non-B
Liver infection caused by viruses other than
hepatitis A and B. Group includes hepatitis C,
hepatitis D and hepatitis E.
(*see HCV, Hep C*)

NB

Nota bene
Note well.

NBI

No bony injury
No evidence of fracture evident on
examination or radiography.
NFS

NBL

Neuroblastoma
Malignant tumour originating from neural
crest cells affecting infants and children.

NBM

Nil by mouth
No fluids or solids to be taken orally.
NPO

NBTNF

Newborn term normal female
Healthy female infant.

NBTNM

Newborn term normal male
Healthy male infant.

NBTS

National Blood Transfusion Service
Agency for the collection and provision of
blood and blood products.

NCBI

**National Centre for Biotechnology
Information**
American body responsible for developing
resources related to research on the human
genome.

NCL

Neuronal ceroid-lipofuscinosis
Clinically heterogeneous group of inherited
neurodegenerative disorders.

NCRP

**National Council on Radiation Protection
and Measurements**
US national advisory body on radiation
protection.

ND

Neoplastic disease
New and abnormal growth of cells in a benign
or malignant tumour. Often used as a
euphemism for cancer.
Neo., NG, Tu

ND

No data

ND

Not detected

ND

Not done

NE tumour

Neuroendocrine tumour
Tumour secreting peptide(s), with
endocrine/neurotransmitter properties.

NEC

Necrotizing enterocolitis
Inflammatory disorder of the neonatal small
intestine of unknown aetiology; causes a
breakdown of the barrier to invasion by
intestinal flora. Gas may then accumulate in
the bowel wall, possibly resulting in
perforation.

NECT

Non-enhanced computerized tomography
Computerized tomography (CT) studies
undertaken without the use of a contrast
agent.

NED

No evidence of disease
Usually means free of local or metastatic
disease after cancer treatment.
NSR, NSR/M

NEFA

Non-esterified fatty acids
Molecule which forms triglyceride lipids when
esterified to glycol. In blood they circulate
bound to albumin providing an important
aerobic source of energy.
FFA

NEJM

New England Journal of Medicine
Premier peer–reviewed weekly medical
journal.
N Engl J Med

NEMA

National Electric Manufacturers Association
Body responsible for setting electrical
standards

N Engl J Med
New England Journal of Medicine
See under NEJM.

Neo.
Neoplasm
See under ND.
NG, Tu.

(The) Net
The Internet (internetworking protocol)
A worldwide system linking smaller computer
networks together, allowing information to be
exchanged between any of their computers.

NET
Neuroendocrine tumour
Malignancy arising from cells of neural crest
origin.
(*see PNET*)

NFR
Not for resuscitation
Patient on whom emergency reanimation will
not be attempted in the event of cardiac or
respiratory arrest.

NFS
No fracture seen
See under NBI.

Ng
Neisseria gonorrhoeae
Gram-negative bacterium responsible for a
sexually transmitted disease (gonorrhoea/
'clap').
GC

NG
Neoplastic growth
See under ND.
Neo, Tu.

NGT
Nasogastric tube
Tube passed through the nose into the
stomach for drainage, lavage or feeding.
NG tube

NG tube
Nasogastric tube
See under NGT.

NGU
Non-gonococcal urethritis
Sexually transmitted urethritis, not caused by
gonococcal infection.

N(H) weighted
Hydrogen density
Magnetic resonance image in which
differences in hydrogen (proton) density are
the major source of image contrast.
Proton density

NHL
Non-Hodgkin's lymphoma
Neoplastic disease of lymphoid tissue
characterized by the presence of the
Reed–Sternberg cell.

NHS
National Health Service
British public health system.

NIC
Network information centre
Place where information about that particular
network is located.

NICER
**Nycomed Intercontinental Continuing
Education in Radiology**
Radiological educational body focusing on
developing countries.

NICU
Neonatal intensive care unit
Ward for premature and sick newborn babies.
NNU, SCBU

NIDDM
Non-insulin dependent diabetes mellitus
Form of diabetes mellitus (DM) which may be
controlled by diet or by drugs that lower the
blood sugar.
(*see IDDM*)

NIDDY
Non-insulin dependent diabetes in the young
Form of diabetes mellitus (DM) occurring in
young people which may be controlled by diet
or by drugs that lower blood sugar. Tends to be
strongly familial.
MODY (obsolete)
(*see IDDM, NIDDM*)

N loop
N-shaped loop
Anatomical configuration of the sigmoid colon
that hinders endoscopy.

nm
Nanometre
10^{-9} m.
(*see m*)

NM (US: NUCS)

Nuclear medicine
Physiological and anatomical imaging using radioactive tracers.
Nuc. med.

NMJ

Neuromuscular junction
Connection between nerve endings and muscles where the neurotransmitter is acetylcholine (Ach).

NMR

Nuclear magnetic resonance
Imaging technique in which images are formed by applying a radiofrequency pulse to a subject in a magnetic field.
MR, MRI

NMRS

Nuclear magnetic resonance spectroscopy
Use of magnetic resonance to obtain spectral information from specific chemical entities in compounds or tissues in the form of peaks analysed according to their frequency, amplitude and area under the peak.
MRS

NN/LM

National network of libraries in medicine
Lists medically related resources available on the Internet.

NNU

Neonatal unit
Ward for premature and sick newborn babies.
NICU, SCBU

NOE

Nuclear Overhauser effect
Change in steady state magnetization of a particular nucleus resulting in irradiation of a neighbouring nucleus with which it is coupled through a spin–spin interaction.

NOF

Neck of femur
Anatomical connection between the head and shaft of the femur.

^{59}NP

p-Iodomethylnorcholesterol
Tracer labelled with iodine-131 (^{131}I) or selenium-75 (^{75}Se) used in nuclear medicine for imaging the adrenal cortex.

NP

Necrotizing pancreatitis
Severe inflammation of the pancreas with associated autolysis.

NPD

Niemann Pick disease
Inborn error of sphingomyelin metabolism causing hepatosplenomegaly and physical and mental retardation.

NPH

Normal pressure hydrocephalus
Syndrome comprising the clinical triad of dementia, apraxia and urinary incontinence. Radiologically the cerebral ventricles are enlarged without cortical atrophy.

NPH

Nucleus pulposus herniation
Protrusion of the central part of an intervertebral disc which, when occurring posteriorly, may impinge on nerve roots resulting in pain or neurological symptoms.

NPO

Nil per oram
See under NBM.

NR

Normal range
Reference interval.

NRC

Nuclear Regulatory Commission
US authority responsible for radiation protection and the safety of radiopharmaceuticals.

NRPB

National Radiation Protection Board
British national advisory body on radiation protection.

NS

Nephrotic syndrome
Kidney disease characterized by albuminuria, hypoalbuminaemia, hyperlipoproteinaemia, and oedema.

NS

Normal saline
See under N saline.

NS

Not significant
Denotes the statistically insignificant result of a scientific study with a p value of >0.05 (usually).

NSA
Number of signals averaged
Number of magnetic resonance (MR) signals averaged together to determine each distinct position. Encoded signal to be used in image construction.

NSAID(s)
Nonsteroidal anti-inflammatory drug(s)
One of a large group of drugs with anti-inflammatory properties, e.g. aspirin.

NSCA
National Center for Supercomputing Applications
US government funded organization to provide high technology resources for the scientific community.

NSCCL
Non-small cell carcinoma of lung
Group of malignant lung tumours, histologically separate from 'oat cell' carcinoma.

NSR
No sign of recurrence
See under NED.

NSR
Normal sinus rhythm
Normal regular beating of the heart.

NSR/M
No sign of recurrence or metastases
See under NED.

NST
Non-stress test
Ultrasound monitoring of fetal heart rate in response to fetal movement. Forms part of the biophysical profile.

NSU
Non-specific urethritis
See under NGU.

NTD
Neural tube defect
Embryonic maldevelopment of the neural tube resulting in cranio–spinal defects, e.g. spina bifida.

NTP
Normal temperature and pressure
Old abbreviation for standard temperature and pressure (STP).

NTSC
National Television Standards Committee
Defines video standard used in USA.

Nucs (US)
Nuclear medicine
See under NM.
Nuc. med.

Nuc. med. (US: Nucs)
Nuclear medicine
See under NM.

N&V
Nausea and vomiting
Feeling and being sick (emesis).

NVD
Normal vaginal delivery
Normal delivery of baby via the vagina.
SD, SVD

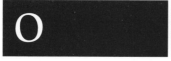

O

Oxygen
Element that is essential to life processes in the animal kingdom.
O_2

O_2

Oxygen
Gaseous molecule essential for respiration.

^{15}O

Oxygen-15
Short-lived beta-emitting radionuclide used in positron emission tomography (PET).
15-O
(see β^+ emission)

OA

Occipitoanterior
One of the possible positions of the fetal head during a vaginal delivery.

OA

Oesophageal atresia
Non-patent oesophageal segment, a developmental defect.
(see TOF)

OA

Osteoarthritis
Degenerative joint disease.

OAF

Osteoclast activity factor(s)
Factor inducing activity of bone resorbing cells.
OSF

Obs.

Observations
Routine observation of vital signs.
TPR

Obs.

Obsolete
No longer used, old-fashioned.

Obs.

Obstetrics
Branch of medicine and surgery which is related to pregnancy and childbirth.

Obs & Gobs

Obstetrics and gynaecology
Medical slang for obstetrics and gynaecology.
O & G, Obs. & Gynae.

Obs. & Gynae.

Obstetrics and gynaecology
Branch of medicine which specializes in pregnancy, childbirth and diseases of women.
O&G, Obs & Gobs

OB-US

Obstetrical ultrasound
Study of the fetus in utero using ultrasound.

OCG

Oral cholecystogram
Imaging of the gall bladder and common bile duct using an oral contrast agent.

OCLC

Online computer library center
US online cooperative cataloguing service.

OC&P

Ova cysts and parasites
Pathogens which are found in tissue or body fluid samples; they often complete their life cycle outside human hosts.
(see O & P)

OCP

Oral contraceptive pill
An oral preparation for contraception. Provides cyclical hormone administration (usually a combination of oestrogen and progesterone) which is aimed at preventing ovulation.

OCR

Optical character recognition
Algorithms that analyse an image by allocating probabilities to each of a set of characters.

OCRS

Oculocerebral renal syndrome
X-linked recessive disorder of amino acid transport. Characterized by congenital ocular abnormalities, mental retardation, renal tubular acidosis, and metabolic bone disease. Lowe syndrome.

od

Once daily
From Latin 'omni die'. Administration (of a drug) once a day.
sid

OD
Optical density
Measure of the blackness of radiographic film.
$D = \lg Io/I$ (Io = incident light intensity;
I = intensity of light transmitted through film).
D

OD
Optical disc
A long-term archive medium. Laser energy is
used to store and retrieve digital data, which
are irreversibly engraved on each disc.

OD
Overdose
Administration of an excessive amount of
drugs (usually self-inflicted).

ODA
Operating department assistant
Health-care worker who assists in the
operating department and anaesthetic room.

ODJ
Optical disc jukebox
Archive for long-term digital image storage.
LTA, LTS

ODQ
On direct questioning
Symptoms to which a patient admits when
asked, but which are not volunteered.
(*see FE, ROS, SE, SR*)

O/E
On examination
Indicates the findings of a physical
examination.
OE

OE
On examination
See under O/E.

OE
Otitis externa
Inflammation of the ear external to the
tympanic membrane.
(*see AO, EAC, EAM*)

OF
Occipito frontal
From the base of the skull to the forehead.
Defines the path of an X-ray beam from tube
to cassette.

OFD
Object film distance
Distance between a radiographic subject and
the film or cassette.
d

O&G
Obstetrics and gynaecology
See under Obs. & gynae.
Obs & Gobs

OGC
Oculo-gyric crisis
Drug-induced acute dystonic reaction which
paralyses the ocular muscles. Can occur with
metoclopramide.

OGD
Oesophago-gastro duodenoscopy
Endoscopic examination of the oesophagus,
stomach and duodenum.

OGJ
Oesophago-gastric junction
Anatomical boundary between the oesophagus
and stomach.

OGTT
Oral glucose tolerance test
Investigation to assess disorders of glucose
metabolism by measuring the blood glucose
response to a glucose meal.
GTT

$1,25-(OH)_2D_3$, 1,25 DACC
Dehydroepiandrosterone
Active metabolite of vitamin D.
(*see CC*)

OHL
Oral hairy leukoplakia
White patches in the mouth which cannot be
removed. Premalignant in 5% of cases.

OHSS
Ovarian hyperstimulation syndrome
Enlarged ovaries with multiple follicular cysts
in patients who are undergoing human
chorionic gonadotrophin (HCG) therapy for
infertility.

OI
Opportunistic infecton
Infectious disease occurring in an
immunocompromised patient which would
not normally cause illness in an
immunocompetent individual.

OIH
Orthoiodohippurate (hippuran)
Tracer labelled with iodine isotopes used in
renal imaging.

OKA
Otherwise known as
(*see AKA*)

OLB
Open lung biopsy
Surgical operation to remove a sample of lung for histological examination.

OM
Once in the morning
From latin 'omni mane.' Administration (of a drug) once in the morning.

OM
Obtuse marginal
Branch of the main circumflex coronary artery. (*see PLCx*)

OM
Occipito mental
From the base of the skull to the chin. Defines the path of an X-ray beam from tube to cassette.

OML
Orbito meatal line
Theoretical line which joins the outer canthus of the eye to the external auditory meatus. Used in positioning for skull radiography.

on
Once at night
From Latin 'omni nocte'. Administration (of a drug) once at night.

ON
Osteonecrosis
Avascular necrosis (AVN) of bone. Bone death occurs as a result of an interruption of its blood supply.

O&P
Ova and parasites
See under OC & P.

O/P, OP
Outpatient
Patient under the care of, but not admitted to, a hospital or clinic.

OP
Occipitoposterior
One of the possible positions of the fetal head during a vaginal delivery.

OPC
Outpatient clinic
Hospital clinic for seeing patients who are not currently resident in that hospital.

OPCA
Olivopontocerebellar atrophy
Neurodegenerative disease which is characterized by atrophy of the olive pons, middle cerebellar peduncles, and cerebellar hemispheres.
OPCD

OPCD
Olivopontocerebellar degeneration
See under OPCA.

op. cit.
opere citato
Latin for: 'in the work cited'. Textual annotation.

OPD
Outpatient department
See under OPC.

OPG
Orthopantomogram
Tomographic radiograph of teeth and jaws.

OPV
Oral poliomyelitis vaccine
Immunization given to children during the first year of life with a booster at school entry and every 10 years thereafter.

OR
Operating room
Operating theatre.

ORh⁻
Blood group O, rhesus negative
Universal donor blood which can safely be given to a person of any blood group without causing an immune reaction.

ORIF
Open reduction internal fixation
Surgical treatment for fractures, involving the internal stabilization of a fracture aligned at operation.
IF

ORS
Oral rehydration salts
Fluid containing sodium, potassium and glucose which is rapidly absorbed. Used in the treatment of diarrhoeal disease to restore the fluid balance.

ORT
Oral rehydration therapy
See under ORS.

OS

Osteosarcoma
Commonest primary malignant tumour of bone.

OSA

Obstructive sleep apnoea
Upper airway occlusion during sleep which causes progressive apnoea until waking occurs. Pickwickian syndrome.

OSF

Osteoclast stimulating factor(s)
See under OAF.

OSI

Open systems interconnection
Seven layer model communications network linking computer systems both within and between organizations, irrespective of the type of computer systems involved.

OT

Occupational therapist
Health care professional involved in practical rehabilitation of patients with disabilities.

OTC

Over the counter
Medicines available without a prescription.

OTM

Oxford Textbook of Medicine
Popular general medical text.

OWR

Osler–Weber–Rendu
Autosomal dominant disorder causing spider naevi in the skin, gastrointestinal tract which may bleed and pulmonary arteriovenous malformations.
HHT
(*see PAVM*)

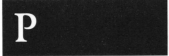

π

Pi
Mathematical constant of the ratio of the circumference of any circle to its diameter.
$\pi = 3.14153962$.

p (value)

Probability value
Statistical likelihood, expressed as a fraction of 1, that a particular observation/result would occur merely by chance. A value of $p < 0.05$ is usually considered to be statistically significant.

P

Para
Number of pregnancies a woman has carried to beyond 28 weeks gestation.

P

Pressure
Force acting on unit area.

P₂

Pulmonary valve component of 2nd heart sound.

PA

Pernicious anaemia
Megaloblastic anaemia, caused by vitamin B12 deficiency as a result of lack of gastric intrinsic factor IF.
(see RAEB)

PA

Postero anterior
From back to front. Defines the direction of an X-ray beam towards a cassette or a film.
(see AP)

PA

Pulmonary artery
Main artery supplying deoxygenated blood to the lungs.

Pa

Pascal
SI unit of pressure. 1 Pa = 1 newton/metre^2 (m).
(see mmHg)

PAB

Premature atrial beat
Early contraction of the atrial chamber, the most frequent benign cardiac arrhythmia in the fetus.
PAC

PAC

Premature atrial contraction
See under PAB.

paCO₂

Arterial partial pressure of carbon dioxide
Biochemical estimation of arterial carbon dioxide level.
pCO_2

PACS

Picture archiving and communications system
A hospital-wide network for generating, viewing, archiving and retrieving digital images and their associated reports.
IMACS
(see HIS, MDIS, RIS)

PACWP

Pulmonary arterial capillary wedge pressure
Pressure-reading which indirectly measures left atrial pressure; obtained by measuring the pressure distal to an occluding balloon in a medium-sized pulmonary artery.
PAWP, PCWP, PWP

Paeds

Paediatrics (U.S. Pedi)
The specialty of diseases of children.

PAF

Plain abdominal film
Frontal abdominal X-ray.
AXR
(see KUB)

PAH

Primary alveolar hypoventilation
Disorder of unknown aetiology, characterized by chronic hypercapnia and hypoxaemia in the absence of identifiable neuromuscular disease.

PAH

Pulmonary arterial hypertension
Pulmonary arterial pressure greater than 30 mmHg in systole. May be primary, or secondary, e.g. to chronic lung disease or intracardiac shunt.

PAL
Phase alternating line
Defines video standard used in Europe (except France).

PAN
Polyarteritis nodosa
Multisystem necrotizing vasculitis of small and medium-sized arteries; microaneurysms of renal and visceral arteries are characteristic.

Panc.
Pancreas
Central abdominal organ with endocrine and exocrine functions; secretions include insulin and digestive enzymes.

paO₂
Arterial partial pressure of oxygen
Biochemical estimation of arterial oxygen level.
pO2

PAP
Primary atypical pneumonia
Nonbacterial pneumonia often caused by *Mycoplasma pneumoniae*.

PAP
Pulmonary alveolar proteinosis
Lung disease of unknown aetiology in which phospholipid accumulates in the alveoli. Treated by bronchoalveolar lavage (BAL).

PAPVC
Partial anomalous pulmonary venous connection
One or more pulmonary veins drain into the right atrium (or superior or inferior vena cava). May be associated with hypogenetic lung syndrome.
PAPVD, PAPVR
(see APVR, HAPVC, HAPVD, HAPVR)

PAPVD
Partial anomalous pulmonary venous drainage
See under PAPVC.
PAPVR
(see APVR, HAPVC, HAPVD, HAPVR)

PAPVR
Partial anomalous pulmonary venous return
See under PAPVC.
PAPVD
(see APVR, HAPVC, HAPVD, HAPVR)

PAS
Periodic acid Schiff
Stain used in histopathology to demonstrate glycosaminoglycan-containing cells.

pat
Patient

Path.
Pathology
1. Branch of medicine concerned with the cause and nature of disease.
2. Manifestations of disease in tissues or organs.
3. Hospital department in which pathology services are located.
Pathol.

PAVM
Pulmonary arteriovenous malformation
Congenital shunt lesion with arterial and venous component(s) in lung. Commonly associated with hereditary haemorrhagic telangiectasia (HHT).
(see OWR)

PAWP
Pulmonary arterial wedge pressure
See under PACWP.
PCWP, PWP

Pb
Lead
Metal commonly used for X-ray shielding and other forms of radiation protection.

PBC
Primary biliary cirrhosis
Chronic progressive bile duct destruction, eventually leading to cirrhosis. Probably has immunological aetiology.

PBG
Porphobilinogen
Precursor in haem pathway. Acts as a urinary marker for acute intermittent porphyria (AIP).

PBPV
Percutaneous balloon pulmonary valvuloplasty
Balloon dilatation of pulmonary valve stenosis using percutaneous approach.

p.c.
Post cibum
After meals (after food).
Post prand.

PC
Personal computer
A computer for individual use, originally
designed and made by IBM.

p/c
Presenting complaint
Main symptom which caused a patient to
consult a doctor.
c/o, PC

PC
Phase contrast
Technique used in magnetic resonance
angiography (MRA).

PC
Politically correct
Forms of English usage regarded as acceptable
by certain pressure groups (especially in the
USA).

PC
Portocaval
Link between portal venous and systemic
venous circulation. Shunts of this type
are used in the treatment of portal
hypertension.

PC
Presenting complaint
See under p/c.
c/o

PCA
Patient-controlled analgesia
Intravenous bolus infusion of (narcotic)
analgesia controlled by patient so that the dose
can be suited to the level of pain.
(see SAM)

PCA
Posterior cerebral artery
Main terminal branch of the basilar artery
supplying the occipital cerebral lobe.

PCB
Post-coital bleeding
Abnormal bleeding *per vaginam* following
sexual intercourse.

PCC
Phaeochromocytoma
Adrenal medullary tumour causing excess
catecholamine secretion with resultant
hypertension.

PCG
Pancreaticocholangiography
Contrast examination of biliary and pancreatic
ducts.

PCKD
Polycystic kidney disease
Autosomal-dominant hereditary disease
causing renal parenchymal cyst formation and
ultimately renal failure. Associated with
pancreatic, splenic and hepatic cysts and
intracranial aneurysms. Usually presents in
adult life.
ADPD, APCD, APD, APKD

PCL
Posterior cruciate ligament
Central knee ligament between femur and
tibia which contributes to joint stability.
(see ACL)

PCM
Protein calorie malnutrition
Physical effects of starvation due to insufficient
protein.

PCMCIA
**Personal computer memory card
international association**
Used to describe computer and technical
equipment that conforms to the credit card
format.

PCO
Polycystic ovarian syndrome
Clinical syndrome of hirsutism, obesity, and
oligomenorrhoea: ultrasound may corroborate
the diagnosis.
PCOD, PCOS

pCO$_2$
Arterial partial pressure of carbon dioxide
See under paCO$_2$.

PCOD
Polycystic ovarian disease
See under PCO.
PCOS

PCOM
Posterior communicating artery
Artery connecting the internal carotid artery
(ICA) and the posterior cerebral artery (PCA)
on each side, forming part of the circle of
Willis.

PCOS
Polycystic ovarian syndrome
See under PCO.
PCOD

PCP
Pneumocystis carinii pneumonia
Opportunistic infection occurring in
immunosuppressed individuals.
(*see AIDS*)

PCR
Polymerase chain reaction
Part of technique for localizing the position of
a gene on a chromosome.

PCRV
Polycythaemia rubra vera
Myeloproliferative disorder causing an increase
in packed red cell volume, with variable
leucocytosis, thrombocythaemia and
splenomegaly.
PCV

PC shunt
Portocaval shunt
Communication between portal venous and
systemic venous circulations. Used in the
treatment of portal hypertension.

PCT
Porphyria cutanea tarda
Uroporphyrin decarboxylase deficiency
causing light-induced blisters,
hyperpigmentation, hirsutism, diabetes and
liver neoplasms.
HP

PCT
Proximal convoluted tubule
Part of the nephron; the major site of
reabsorption of salt and water.

PCV
Packed cell volume
That volume of blood which is composed of
red blood cells.

PCV
Polycythemia vera
See under PCRV.

PCWP
Pulmonary capillary wedge pressure
See under PACWP.
PAWP, PWP

PD
Parkinson's disease
Neurodegenerative disease characterized
clinically by resting 'pill-rolling' tremor,
rigidity and bradykinesia. There is generation
of pigmented neurones in the substantia nigra
and other brain stem nuclei.

PD
Peritoneal dialysis
Renal replacement therapy allowing the
excretion of metabolic waste across the
peritoneum into the peritoneal fluid which is
exchanged regularly via a permanent catheter.

PD
Pick's disease
Cortical dementia, commonly of presenile
onset. Characteristic neuropathological
markers and striking lobar atrophy (frontal,
temporal) are features of the disorder.

PD
Posterior descending
Terminal branch of the right coronary artery.

PD
Potential difference
Difference in electrical potential between two
points.

PD
Pancreatic duct
Central draining vessel of the pancreas,
emptying into the duodenum via the ampulla
of Vater.
MPD

PDA
Patent ductus arteriosus
Persistent fetal connection between the main
pulmonary artery and the aorta, causing left to
right shunt.
(*see DA*)

PDGF
Platelet derived growth factor
Agent released by normal blood vessels in
response to vessel injury.

PDN
Public data network
Network leased from telecommunications
companies, used to transmit data outside the
hospital/institution.

PDPDM

Protein-deficient pancreatic diabetes mellitus
Diabetes mellitus (DM) occurring in association with malnutrition and low body weight.

PDQ

Pretty damn(ed) quick
Urgent.
(see ASAP)

PDS

Personal display station
A workstation with monitors for showing radiological images. May be part of a picture archiving and communication system (PACS).

PDS

Penile Doppler studies
Ultrasound assessment of the penile vascular supply.

PE

Pulmonary embolism/embolus/emboli
Occlusion of the pulmonary artery or its branches usually by thrombus arising at a distant site.

PE segment

Pharyngoesophageal segment
Upper portion of the gastrointestinal tract (GIT) and its associated muscles, extending from the back of the oral cavity to the upper oesophageal sphincter.

PED

Patient evaluation by doctor
Medical assessment of a patient's well-being and progress.

PEEP

Positive end expiratory pressure
Technique used in mechanical ventilation to maintain positive pressure in the alveoli at the end of expiration.

PEFR

Peak expiratory flow rate
Maximum flow of air generated by forced exhalation. Used in the evaluation of 'obstructive' lung disease.

PEG

Percutaneous endoscopic gastrostomy
Endoscopic technique used to introduce a feeding tube into the stomach.

PEG

Pneumoencephalography
Obsolete technique for imaging the ventricles of the brain using air as the contrast medium.

PEJ

Percutaneous endoscopic jejunostomy
Endoscopic technique used to introduce a feeding tube into the proximal small bowel.

PEL

Permissible exposure limits
Maximum dose of ionizing radiation to which an individual may be exposed during a stated time.

PEM

Protein energy malnutrition
Starvation.

PERLA

Pupils equal and reactive to light and accommodation
Describes intact pupillary reflexes.

PET

Positron emission tomography
Cross-sectional functional imaging based on positron-emitting radionuclides.

PET

Pre-eclamptic toxaemia
Hypertension in pregnancy with associated proteinuria and/or oedema.

Pex

Peak exercise
The limit of exercise tolerance, usually on a treadmill or bicycle.

PFO

Patent foramen ovale
Atrial septal defect caused by failure of normal closure of the foramen ovale at birth.

PFT

Pulmonary function tests
Respiratory assessment based on spirometric testing.
LFT, RFT

PGI$_2$

Prostacyclin
Factor produced by endothelial cells from arachidonic acid. It blocks platelet activation and aggregation, and promotes vasodilatation.

PGL

Persistent generalized lymphadenopathy
Lymph nodes greater than 1 cm diameter in at least two non-inguinal sites persisting for at least three months with no known cause. Associated with human immunodeficiency virus (HIV) infection.

PH
Past history
Previous illnesses or operations.
PMH

pH
Logarithmic expression of hydrogen ion concentration on a scale of 1 (acid) to 14 (alkaline). Measure of the acidity or alkalinity of a solution.

PHA
Pulse height analyser
Component of a gamma camera that selects signals from primary photons and discards signals from scattered ones.

PhD
Doctor of Philosophy
Academic post-graduate degree requiring several years of research.
(see MD)

PHP
Pseudohypoparathyroidism
Hereditary disorder characterized by the symptoms and signs of hypoparathyroidism associated with distinctive skeletal defects, such as a short fourth metacarpal.

pHPT
Primary hyperparathyroidism
Elevation of the parathyroid hormone (PTH) due to a secreting parathyroid tumour.
1° HPT

p.i.
Post injection
After injection.

PI
Pulmonary incompetence
Leaky pulmonary valve.
PR

PI
Pulsatility index
Difference between maximum and minimum Doppler shift frequencies divided by the time averaged mean. Indicates the pulsatility of a vessel independent of the angle between the ultrasound beam and the vessel wall.

PICA
Posterior inferior cerebellar artery
Branch of the vertebral artery supplying the lower cerebellum.

PID
Picture image directory
Series of miniature token images in a picture archiving and communication system (PACS).

PID
Pelvic inflammatory disease
Infection of the female genital tract.

PID
Prolapsed intervertebral disc
'Slipped disc', usually posteriorly, causing impingement of the intervertebral disc on the thecal sac or exiting nerve roots.

PIE
Pulmonary infiltrate with eosinophilia
Infiltration of the lung with eosinophils which may be idiopathic or due to various causes, e.g. parasitic infestation, drugs.

PIE
Pulmonary interstitial emphysema
Gas in the mediastinum and interstitial tissues of the lung, usually emanating from a bronchial or alveolar leak. Possible sequel to respiratory distress syndrome (RDS) in premature infants.

PIF
Prolactin-release inhibiting factor
Dopamine. Inhibits the release of prolactin.

PIH
Prolactin-inhibiting hormone
See under PIF.

PIIS
Posterior inferior iliac spine
Bony protuberance on the lower part of the back of the iliac bone.

PIOPED
Prospective investigation of pulmonary embolism diagnosis
Large American study on the diagnosis of pulmonary embolism (PE) with ventilation perfusion scans (V/Q scan) performed in 1983. It states the criteria for diagnosing low, intermediate and high probability of PE.

PIPJ
Proximal interphalangeal joint
Synovial joint between the proximal and middle phalanges of the hand or foot.

Pit.
Pituitary
Gland inferior to the third ventricle lying in the pituitary fossa, it secretes hormones which mostly regulate the release of other hormones.

Pixel
Picture element
The smallest part of an image. It is assigned one of a range of grey levels or colours.

PK
Pyruvate kinase
Enzyme which catalyses the last step in the glycolytic pathway. Deficient in a group of inherited red cell disorders.

PKU
Phenylketonuria
Inherited disorder of amino acid metabolism which leads to an accumulation of phenylalanine in blood and urine. If untreated it leads to devastating mental retardation.

PL
Prolactin
Hormone released by the anterior pituitary which stimulates milk production.
PRL

Plat.
Platelets
Mega karyocyte cell fragments essential for normal clotting mechanisms.
P'lets, Plts

PLCx
Posterolateral circumflex branches
Branches of the main circumflex coronary artery.
(*see* OM)

P'lets
Platelets
See under Plat.
Plts

PLP
Posterior lobe of pituitary
One of the two lobes of the pituitary gland.
Post. pit.
(*see* ALP)

Plts
See under Plat.
P'lets

PM
Pacemaker
Internal or external electrical device with wires to the heart chambers that maintains an adequate heart rate.
(*see* PPM)

PM
Polymyositis
Generalized inflammatory disorder of muscle.

pm
Premolar
Tooth, for chewing. There are a total of eight in humans, each pair lying between the canine and molar teeth.

PMB
Post-menopausal bleeding
Bleeding *per vaginam* (PV) following the menopause.

PMC
Pseudomembranous colitis
Diarrhoeal illness following use of broad spectrum antibiotics, associated with strains of *Clostridium difficile*.
AAC, AAPC

PMF
Progressive massive fibrosis
Pneumoconiosis complicated by lung fibrosis which may continue to progress after the cessation of dust exposure.

PMH
Past medical history
See under PH.

PML
Posterior mitral leaflet
One of the two leaflets of the mitral valve.
pMVL

PML
Progressive multifocal leucoencephalopathy
Viral infection of immunocompromised patients leading to extensive white matter demyelination, with relative sparing of cortical grey matter.

PMN
Polymorphonuclear leucocyte / neutrophil
Type of white blood cell with a multilobular nucleus.

PMR
Polymyalgia rheumatica
Inflammatory disorder of proximal muscles associated with markedly elevated erythrocyte sedimentation rate (ESR).

pMVL
Posterior mitral valve leaflet
See under PML.

PN
Postnatal
Period following birth.

PNA
Partial nail ablation
Surgical removal of part of the nail bed as a treatment for in-growing toe nail.

PND
Paroxysmal nocturnal dyspnoea
Awakening from sleep with difficulty in breathing. Symptom of poorly controlled left ventricular failure (LVF).

PND
Post-nasal drip
Symptom of persistent secretion into the nasopharynx.

PNET
Primitive neuroectodermal tumour
A central nervous system tumour arising from a primitive cell line containing cells capable of differentiating into medulloblasts, astrocytes, oligodendrocytes, ependyma, ganglion cells or skeletal muscle.

PNH
Paroxysmal nocturnal haemoglobinuria
Haemolytic anaemia, often of the young, characterized by intermittent haemoglobinuria, mild granulocytopenia, and thrombocytopenia.

PNS
Parasympathetic nervous system
Part of the nervous system controlling visceral functions of the body. Uses acetylcholine (Ach) as a neurotransmitter in the post-ganglionic neurons.

PNS
Peripheral nervous system
Nervous system outside the brain and spinal cord.

Pnthx
Pneumothorax
Accumulation of air (or any gas) in the pleural space.
Px

po
per orem
By mouth.

pO$_2$
Arterial partial pressure of oxygen
See under paO$_2$.

PO$_4{}^{2-}$
Phosphate
Salt of phosphoric acid. A constituent of human bones. Also found in the blood, where it can be measured.

POBA
Plain old balloon angioplasty
Balloon dilatation of a vascular stenosis using a catheter inserted through the skin at a site distant from the stenosis.

POD
Pouch of Douglas
Peritoneal recess between the bladder and rectum.

POEMS
Polyneuropathy, organomegaly, endocrinopathy, M protein, skin changes
Syndrome characterized by the above symptoms.

POETS
Push off early; tomorrow is Saturday
Hospital euphenism for leaving duty early on Friday afternoon.

Polio.
Poliomyelitis
Viral inflammation of the anterior horn cells of the spinal cord and cranial nerve nuclei, commonly resulting in motor paralysis.

POM
Prescription only medicine
Drug or medical preparation available only when ordered by a doctor or dentist.

POMP
Phase-offset multiplanar
Pulse sequence in magnetic resonance imaging that doubles the number of slices per repetition time.

POP

Plaster of Paris
Gypsum (calcium sulphate) cast used to immobilize fractures.

POP

Progestogerone only pill
A contraceptive tablet consisting only of progestogens which prevent fertilization and implantation.

post./POST.

Posterior
Used in anatomical descriptions to denote dorsal situation; 'behind'.
(see ant, inf., sup.)

POST

Power-on self-test
The first thing a personal computer (PC) does after switching on: checks that all hardware components are running and that the central processing unit (CPU) and memory are functioning properly.

Post-op (US: S/P)

Post operative / operation
Following an operation.

Post. pit.

Posterior pituitary
See under PLP.
(see ant. pit.)

Post prand.

Post prandium
After a meal.

Post. tib.

Posterior tibial
Anatomical description for the compartment, vessels and nerve of the back of the lower leg.

POTS

Plain old telephone service
Data transmission over a good quality voice-grade telephone line, supporting a rate of 19.2 kbits/s (19,200 baud).

PP

Postpartum
The immediate time period following childbirth.

PP

Private patient
Patient whose medical expenses are not met by the National Health Service.

PPF

Plasma protein fraction/purified plasma protein
Isotonic solution containing protein, mostly albumin, derived from plasma or serum. Used in hypoproteinaemic conditions of low plasma volume, e.g. burns.

PPG

Photoplethysmography
Method of measuring limb extremity blood flow using a waterbath and light sensor.

PPG

Portal pressure gradient
Parameter used in TIPSS assessment.

PPH

Post-partum haemorrhage
Bleeding following childbirth.

PPHP

Pseudopseudohypoparathyroidism
Hereditary disorder characterized by phenotypic defects similar to pseudohypoparathyroidism but without any associated disorder in calcium metabolism.

PPLO

Pleuropneumonia-like organism
Mycoplasma pneumoniae, an organism causing atypical pneumonia.

PPM

Permanent pacemaker
Electrical device inserted beneath the skin of the anterior thoracic wall, with wires to the heart chambers to maintain an adequate heart rate.
(see PM)

ppm

Parts per million
Unit of concentration (usually with reference to gases).

PPP

Peripheral pulses present
Description used in the clinical assessment of peripheral vascular disease usually with respect to the pedal pulses.

PPP

Photostimulable phosphor plate
Imaging plate used to capture a latent radiographic image, later 'read out' by a laser in computed radiographic digital imaging. It is the equivalent of the film-screen combination in conventional radiography.
IP, PSP

PPPP
Pylorus preserving partial pancreaticoduodenectomy
Operation to remove the head of the pancreas whilst retaining the gastric outlet.

PPS
Post-post-scriptum
Further afterthought.
(see PS)

PR
Per rectum
Via the anus and rectum.
TR

PR
Pulmonary regurgitation
See under PI.

PR imaging
Projection reconstruction imaging
Imaging technique in magnetic resonance in which projection profiles of the body are obtained by observing signals using a set of magnetic gradients aligned at different angles with respect to the imaged object.

PR interval
Period between P and R waves of the cardiac electrical cycle, representing the time lag between atrial depolarization and ventricular contraction.

PRE
Proton relaxation enhancement
Enhancement of the signal intensity of hydrogen spectra or images using contrast agents.

Pre-op
Pre-operative
Prior to a surgical procedure.

PREM
Premature infant
Infant born before expected date of delivery, i.e. after less than 37 weeks gestation.

PRF
Pulse repetition frequency
Rate at which separate bursts of ultrasound waves are emitted from an ultrasound probe.

PRHO
Pre-registration house officer
Most junior hospital doctor.
HO
(see HP, HS)

PRIND
Partially reversible ischaemic neurological deficit
Incompletely reversible ischaemic event resulting in neurological dysfunction lasting longer than 24 hours.
(see CVA, RIND, TIA)

PRL
Prolactin
See under PL.

prn
Pro re nata
As necessary, as required.

PROM
Premature rupture of membrane
Rupture of the amniotic sac before the expected date of delivery of a fetus leading to premature delivery.

PROMIS
Problem-orientated medical information system
Schema for recording patient details based on evaluation of their presenting problems.

prop
Proportional
Used in equations to express the proportionality of physical quantities.
α

PRS
Pierre Robin syndrome
Congenital combination of micrognathia, cleft palate and glossoptosis with or without other associated anomalies.

PRS
Proctorectosigmoidoscopy
Endoscopic examination of the anus, rectum and distal sigmoid colon.

PRV
Polycythaemia rubra vera
A myeloproliferative disorder causing an increase in red cell mass.
PV

PS
Parkinson's syndrome
Neurodegenerative disorder characterized by rigidity, bradykinesia and tremor.

PS
Partial saturation
Magnetic resonance technique of applying repeated radiofrequency pulses with repetition time less than or equal to T_1. Generates images with increased contrast between regions of different T_1.

PS
Pulmonary stenosis
Narrowing of the pulmonary valve: the cardiac valve situated between the right ventricle and the main pulmonary artery.

PS
Post scriptum
Afterthought added at the end of a letter.

PSA
Prostate specific antigen
Protein assayed in the diagnosis and management of prostatic cancer.

PSC
Primary sclerosing cholangitis
Hepatobiliary disorder of unknown aetiology, characterized by progressive biliary fibrosis and ultimately biliary cirrhosis and hepatocellular failure.
SC

PSD
Phase-sensitive detection
Method for balancing real and imaginary channels in magnetic resonance to eliminate any hardware-induced artifacts.

PSE
Present state examination
Standard rating system assessing psychiatric symptoms.

PSF
Point spread function
Mathematical representation of the image produced by a single point of radiation.

PSGN
Poststreptococcal glomerulonephritis
Acute glomerulonephritis (AG) secondary to pharyngeal or cutaneous infection with group A β-haemolytic streptococci.

PSH
Past surgical history
Details of a patient's previous operations and anaesthetics.
SH

PSL
Photostimulable luminescence
Modality using laser-read photostimulable phosphor plates (PSP) to produce hard or soft-copy digital radiographic images.
CR, DR, DLR

PSIS
Posterior superior iliac spine
Bony protuberance on the upper part of the posterior aspect of the iliac bone.

PSM
Pan systolic murmur
Turbulent blood flow audible at the same intensity on auscultation throughout the ventricular contraction, suggestive of atrioventricular valve regurgitation.

PSP
Percutaneous splenoportography
Percutaneous puncture of the spleen with the injection of contrast medium to demonstrate splenic and portal veins.

PSP
Photostimulable phosphor (plate)
See under PPP.
IP

PSP
Progressive supranuclear palsy
Neurodegenerative syndrome of axial rigidity, supranuclear gaze palsy, and pseudobulbar palsy, with marked midbrain and tectal atrophy.

PSS
Progressive systemic sclerosis
Multisystem disorder characterized by fibrosis of the skin, blood vessels and visceral organs such as the gastrointestinal tract, lungs and kidneys. Often associated with the CREST syndrome.
SCD, SS

PSSE
Partial saturation spin echo
Partial saturation technique with repetition time (TR) less than T_1, in which the signal is detected as a spin echo. Used in magnetic resonance imaging (MRI).

PSU
Power supply unit
The part of a desktop computer that converts AC mains voltage down to the low DC voltage used by most computer components.

PSVER
Pattern shift visual evoked responses
Study of electrical activity in the brain in response to specific visual stimuli, recorded by electrodes placed over the posterior portion of the scalp. Often abnormal in optic neuritis, raising suspicion of multiple sclerosis.
VEP, VER

PSVT
Paroxysmal supraventricular tachycardia
Abnormal focus of electrical activity in the atria, or the conducting system above the ventricles, causing intermittent rapid cardiac contractions.
(see SVT)

PT
Parathyroids
Four glands usually lying behind the thyroid which are responsible for the secretion of parathyroid hormone (PTH).

PT
Prothrombin time
Test used in the assessment of blood coagulation status.
PTT

PT
Pyramidal tract
Fasciculus in the central nervous system (CNS).

PTA
Percutaneous transluminal angioplasty
Balloon dilatation of a vascular stenosis using a catheter inserted through the skin at a site distant from the stenosis.
TAP, TLA

PTA
Post-traumatic amnesia
Loss of memory after an accident or stressful life event.

PTBD
Percutaneous transhepatic biliary drainage
Technique in which a catheter is inserted through the skin into the biliary tree to relieve an obstruction.

PTC
Percutaneous transhepatic cholangiography
Contrast examination of the biliary tree achieved by direct puncture of the liver through the skin.

PTCA
Percutaneous transluminal coronary angioplasty
Balloon dilatation of a coronary arterial stenosis using a catheter inserted through the skin at a site distant from the heart.

PTH
Parathyroid hormone
Hormone produced by the parathyroid glands which controls calcium metabolism.

PTO
Please turn over
Textual annotation.

PTT
Partial thromboplastin time
Test used in assessment of blood coagulation status.

PTT
Prothrombin time
See under PT.

PTU
Propylthiouracil
Drug used to treat hyperthyroidism.

PTV
Posterior tibial vein
A vein draining the lower leg.

PU
Peptic ulceration
Ulceration of gastric or duodenal mucosa.
PUD
(see DU, GDU, GU, HP, H. pylori)

PUBS
Percutaneous umbilical blood sampling
Means of obtaining a blood sample from the umbilical cord under ultrasound guidance in a pregnant woman.

PUC
Premature uterine contractions
Abnormal uterine contractions, threatening premature delivery before 37 weeks gestation.

PUD
Peptic ulcer disease
Ulceration of the stomach or duodenum.
PU
(see DU, GDU, GU, HP, H. pylori)

PUJ
Pelvi-ureteric junction
Anatomical boundary between the renal pelvis and proximal ureter.
UPJ

PUJO
Pelvi-ureteric junction obstruction
Outflow obstruction of urine at the
pelvicaliceal junction either intrinsic,
intramural or extrinsic in nature.

PUO
Pyrexia of unknown origin
Persistent fever from an unidentified cause.

PUV
Posterior urethral valves
Obstructive folds of the urethral mucosa
originating from the veru montanum.
A congenital abnormality, commoner
in boys.

PUVA
Psoralen ultraviolet A
Treatment for psoriasis involving a
photosensitizing agent taken orally or topically
and long-wave ultraviolet irradiation.

PV
Per vaginam
Latin for 'through the vagina'. Refers to the
passage of the fetus, fluids, instruments, etc.
In imaging it frequently refers to the mode of
access, e.g. in certain ultrasound examinations.
TV

PV
Polycythaemia vera
See under PRV.

PV
Portal vein
Vein formed by splenic and superior
mesenteric veins which carries visceral blood
to the liver.
HPV, MPV

PV
Pulmonary valve
Heart valve situated between the right
ventricle and pulmonary outflow tract.

PVD
Peripheral vascular disease
Usually refers to atherosclerosis of the
peripheral arterial bed.
(*see* AOD, ASCVD, ASHD, ASPVD)

PVH
Pulmonary venous hypertension
Considered to be present when the pulmonary
capillary wedge pressure (PCWP) is greater
than 15 mmHg. Occurs with left ventricular
inflow tract obstruction or left ventricular
failure.

PVL
Periventricular leucomalacia / leukomalacia
Damage to the white matter of a premature
infant brain, usually secondary to ischaemic
hypoxia.

PVNS
Pigmented villonodular synovitis
Proliferation of joint synovium with
haemosiderin deposition, subchondral erosions
and cystic areas of deossification.

PVR
Peripheral vascular resistance
Opposition to blood flow offered by the entire
systemic vascular tree.
SVR, TPR, TPVR, TSVR, TVR.

PVR
Pulmonary valve replacement / repair
Replacement or repair of the pulmonary valve.

PW
Pulse width
Difference between the systolic and diastolic
pressures.

PWP
Pulmonary wedge pressure
See under PACWP.
PAWP, PCWP

Px
Pneumothorax
See under Pnthx.

PXE
Pseudoxanthoma elasticum
Generalized disorder of the elastic tissue;
affecting skin, eyes and vascular structures.

Pye.
Pyeloplasty
Operation to widen the pelviureteric junction
(PUJ) and thereby relieve an obstruction.

PYP
Pyrophosphate
Tracer labelled with ^{99m}technetium used for
imaging myocardial infarction.

PZT
Lead zirconate titanate
A piezoelectric material used to make
ultrasound transducers.

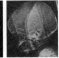

Q factor
In ultrasound the factor relates the operating frequency of the ultrasound probe to the bandwidth, i.e. the range of frequencies involved in a pulse.

Q factor
Quality factor
Weighting factor for individual types of ionizing radiation according to their radiobiological effectiveness (RBE). Used to calculate a comparable quantity, the dose equivalent (H) = QF * absorbed dose (D).
(see Sv)

Q fever
Query fever
Coxiella burnetti infection causing influenza-like illness and atypical pneumonia (rickettsial zoonosis).

QA
Quality assurance
Routine performance checks, e.g. of X-ray equipment ensuring it meets safety specifications and continues to operate at peak performance.
QC

QALY
Quality adjusted life year
Term used in comparing the prognosis of different illnesses using both survival time and assessment of well-being.

QBE
Query by example
Means of interrogating a computer data base to search for a required entity.

QC
Quality control
See under QA.

qds, QDS
quarter die surrendium
To be taken four times a day
qid, QID

QED
quod erat demonstrandum
That which was to have been shown or proved.

QF
Quality factor
See under Q factor.
(see Sv)

qh
quaque hora
Every hour.

qid, QID
quarter in die
See under qds.

QOS
Quality of service
Measure of network uptime.

qqh
quatra quaque hora
From latin for 'every four hours'. To be taken four hourly.

QRS
QRS complex
Electrical activity on an electrocardiogram relating to ventricular contraction.

QT interval
Time between cardiac ventricular depolarization (contraction) and repolarization.

q.v
Latin for: quod vide
Literally; 'which look up'. Refers reader to source material. Textual annotation.

R
Right

R⁺
Rinné positive
Indicates that the the air conduction of sound is better than its bone conduction. Indicates normal hearing or sensorineural hearing loss.

R⁻
Rinné negative
Indicates that the conduction of sound through the bone of the mastoid process is better than its conduction through air. Indicates conductive deafness.

R1
Longitudinal relaxivity or efficiency
Measured per unit concentration of solute of an agent that alters T_1 relaxation rates. Used in magnetic resonance techniques.

R2
Transverse relaxivity or efficiency
Measured per unit concentration of solute of an agent that alters T_2 relaxation rates. Used in magnetic resonance techniques.

r
Grid ratio
Ratio between the height of the lead strips (h) in a grid and the distance between them (D).

r
Physical density
Mass per volume.

r
Radius
Half the diameter of a circle.

R
Resistance
Opposition of a resistor (e.g. wire) to the flow of an electric current (i). Usually ohmic, resistance = voltage (V)/current (i).

R
Roentgen (Röntgen)
Old unit for radiation exposure.
$1 R = 2.58 \times 10^{-4}$ coulomb (C)/kilogram (kg).

RA
Radioactive
Property of a substance undergoing spontaneous disintegration of the nucleus of an atom, with emission of alpha, beta or gamma radiation.

RA
Refractory anaemia
Low haemoglobin resistant to treatment.

RA
Rheumatoid arthritis
Chronic multisystem disorder characterized by symmetrical, inflammatory, peripheral synovitis leading to arthropathy.

RA
Right arm

RA
Right atrial branch
Branch of the right coronary artery.

RA
Right atrium
Right heart chamber which receives blood from the systemic venous system.

RAD
Right axis deviation
Abnormal cardiac electrical vector shown on electrocardiogram (ECG).

RAEB
Refractory anaemia with excess blasts
Megaloblastic anaemia, usually due to vitamin B12 or folate deficiency.
(see IF, PA)

RAID
Redundant array of inexpensive disks
A 'stack' of hard disks operating in parallel so they back each other up if one (or more) fails. Often used for short-term data storage.
(see WSU)

RAM
Random access memory
The local storage area of a computer in which programs and data are held while they are being processed. RAM size is important for the fast manipulation of data, such as images.

RAM-FAST
Reduced acquisition matrix – Fourier acquired steady state
Fast scanning technique in magnetic resonance imaging (MRI).

RAMP

Remote access maintenance protocol
Emerging as standard on the Internet for the
automatic configuration user accounts on
service provider hosts.

RAO

Right anterior oblique
Radiographic projection in which the right
anterior oblique part of the patient is nearest
the cassette film or image-intensifier.

RARE

**Rapid acquisition with relaxation
enhancement**
Multiple spin-echo sequence with echo
encoding, multiple phase steps. Term used
in magnetic resonance imaging (MRI).

RAS

Renal artery stenosis
Narrowing of the renal artery. The condition
may cause hypertension (HT) if severe.

RAST

Radioallergoabsorbent test
Measure of IgE produced in response to a
specific antigen; the IgE is bound to a
small cellulose disc, allowing detection of tiny
quantities of material.

^{81}Rb, Rb-81

Rubidium-81
Radioactive parent of Krypton-81m (81m-Kr)
used in generator.

RB

Right bronchus
Main artery to right lung.
RMB
(see LB, LMB)

RBBB

Right bundle branch block
Impaired conduction of normal cardiac
electrical activity causing abnormal
interventricular depolarization.

RBC

Red blood (cell) count
Quantification of the circulating red blood cell
population.

RBE

Relative biological effectiveness
Relative effect of a certain type of ionizing
radiation on living tissues when compared
with 220 kilovolt peak (kVp) X-rays.
Q

RBL

Radiographic baseline
Theoretical line joining the outer canthus of
the eye with the external auditory meatus.
Used in positioning for skull radiography.
OML

RC

Roman Catholic
Branch of Christianity with administrative
headquarters in the Vatican, which recognizes
the Pope as head of the Christian church.
(see C of E)

RCA

Right coronary artery
Main vessel supplying right ventricle.

rCBV

Regional cerebral blood volume
The volume of blood flowing within a region
of brain tissue.

RCC

Renal cell carcinoma
Malignant tumour of the kidney.
Synonym: hypernephroma (obsolete).

RCM

Right costal margin
Inferior border of the right thoracic cage.

RCR

Royal College of Radiologists
One of two official British
radiological/oncological bodies.
(see BIR)

RCT

Radiotherapy and chemotherapy
Anti-cancer treatment involving use of
therapeutic irradiation and cytotoxic agents.

RCT

Randomized controlled trial
Experimental approach whereby
objects/individuals under study are allocated
at random to one of a defined set of test
conditions.

rd

rad
Non SI unit for absorbed dose (D).
1 rd = 10^{-2} gray (Gy).
(see mrad, mrd)

R&D

Research and development

Experimental investigation, frequently involving a new drug, treatment or technology, often with a view to potential commercial application.

RD

Retinal detachment

Separation of the sensory retina from the retinal pigment epithelium.

RDA

Recommended daily allowance

Quantity of particular nutrient which should be eaten each day as part of a healthy balanced diet.

RDI

RDI

Recommended daily intake

See under RDA.

RDP

Right dextro posterior

Position of the fetus *in utero.*

RDS

Respiratory distress syndrome

Acute respiratory insufficiency in premature neonate due to a lack of surfactant. 'Ground-glass' air-space consolidation is seen on a chest radiograph.

HMD (obsolete)

(see ARDS)

RE

Rectal examination

Digital examination of the anus, rectum and structures palpable through the rectal wall, e.g. prostate.

PR

RED

Rectal evacuatory disorder

Constipation due to a colonic motility disorder.

Reg.

Registrar

Middle grade junior hospital doctor.

REM

Rapid eye movement

Deep sleep associated with rapid eye movement, during which dreaming occurs.

SOREM

RES

Reticuloendothelial system

Group of mononuclear phagocytic cells within different organs.

Resus.

Resuscitation

Reanimation after cardiac or respiratory arrest. (see ECM, NFR)

RF

Releasing factor

Hormone secreted by the hypothalamus acting as a stimulant for a specific anterior pituitary hormone secretion.

RH

RF

Renal failure

Impairment of renal function to a degree that impairs the elimination of toxic metabolic products.

(see ARF, ATN, CRF)

RF

Resonant frequency

Frequency at which protons precess within an applied magnetic field. Equals their Larmor frequency. Magnetic resonance term.

RF

Respiratory failure

Failure adequately to oxygenate the circulating blood.

RF

Rheumatic fever

Inflammatory disease resulting from infection with a group A *Streptococcus* which affects heart, skin, joints and central nervous system (CNS).

Rh F

RF

Rheumatoid factor

Ig M antibody expressed in 80% of patients with rheumatoid arthritis (RA).

RF

Radiofrequency

Transmission in the frequency of radiowaves.

RFC

Request for comments

A series of documents that describe various technical aspects of the Internet.

RFH
Right femoral hernia
Protrusion of abdominal contents into the right femoral canal.

RFLP
Restriction fragment length polymorphism
Part of the technique for localizing the position of a gene on a chromosome.

RF pulse
Radiofrequency pulse
Transmission in the frequency of radiowaves used to alter the orientation of precession of nuclei in magnetic resonance.

RFS
Rotating-frame spectroscopy
Magnetic resonance spectroscopy technique using surface coils taking advantage of spins near the surface.
SCRF

RFT
Respiratory function test
Respiratory assessment based on spirometric testing.
LFTs, PFTs

RGB
Red, green, blue
A colour system that specifies a colour in terms of its proportions of red, green and blue.

RGN
Registered general nurse
Fully qualified nurse.
SRN

RH
Releasing hormone
See under RF.

Rh
Rhenium
Metal added to tungsten (W) in an X-ray tube anode to increase its heat endurance.
(*see* W)

Rh
Rhesus factor
Complex blood group system with antigenic expression, such that individuals with different groups may be immunized by pregnancy or transfusion, with resultant haemolysis or haemolytic disease of the newborn (HDN).

Rh
Rhodium
Metal used for X-ray filtration in mammography (mammo).

RH
Right hand

Rh F
Rheumatic fever
Inflammatory disease resulting from infection with a group A *Streptococcus* which affects the heart, skin, joints and central nervous system (CNS).
RF

RHC
Right hypochondrium
Right subcostal region of the abdomen.

RHF
Right heart failure
Inability of the right ventricle to pump blood adequately resulting in systemic congestion.
RVF
(*see* CCF, CHF, HF, LVF)

RHL
Right hepatic lobe
Anatomical term to describe the part of the liver supplied by the right portal vein and right hepatic arteries.
RLL
(*see* LHL, LLL)

RHR
Resting heart rate
Pulse rate in an individual sitting or lying quietly.

rHuEPO
Recombinant human erythropoietin
Synthetic form of the hormone which regulates red blood cell production. Produced *in vitro* by genetic engineering techniques and is used for the treatment of anaemia in chronic renal failure (CRF).
EPO

RHS
Right hand side
On the right.

RHV
Right hepatic vein
One of the three principal veins draining the liver into the inferior vena cava.

RI
Refractive index
Ratio of the speed of light in a vacuum to the speed of light of the same wavelength in the material under consideration.

RI
Resistive index
Difference between peak systolic and end
diastolic Doppler shift frequencies divided by
the peak systolic. Measures the pulsatility of
flowing vascular beds with no reverse flow
component, e.g. renal.

RIA
Radioimmunoassay
Technique for measuring antibody–antigen
interactions using competition between
radiolabelled and unlabelled antigen for
binding sites on antibodies.

RIA
Reversible ischaemic attack
Episode of pain caused by an insufficient
supply of oxygen to the heart muscle,
not severe enough to cause myocardial
necrosis.

RICU
Respiratory intensive care unit
Ward equipped for the specialist management
of patients in respiratory failure.
(see ICU)

RIF
Radiological interface
The connection between a radiological
information system (RIS) and another
computer network, usually a picture archiving
and communication system (PACS).

RIF
Right iliac fossa
Anatomical term referring to the right lower
abdominal region.

RIH
Right inguinal hernia
Protrusion of abdominal contents into the
right inguinal canal.

RIJ
Right internal jugular
Main vein on the right side of the neck
draining the brain.
(see EJV, Ext Jug V, IJV, Int Jug V, JV,
Jug V, LIJ)

RIMA
Right internal mammary artery
Right anterior chest wall artery used in
coronary arterial bypass surgery.
(see IMA, LIMA)

RIN
Radioisotope nephrography
Imaging of the renal tract using radioisotopes.
Gives both anatomical and functional
information.

RIND
Reversible ischaemic neurological deficit
Fully reversible ischaemic event resulting in
minor neurological dysfunction lasting longer
than 24 hours.
CVA
(see PRIND, TIA)

RIS
Radiology information system
Computerized system which documents the
details of patients attending a radiology
department.

RISC
Reduced instruction set computer
Integrated circuits used in a variety of
computers, communications hardware and
instruments.

RK
Right kidney

R. lat
Right lateral
Radiographic projection in which the right
side of the patient is nearest the film.

RLD
Related live donor
Organ donation from a genetic relative of the
recipient to reduce risk of rejection.

RLF
Retrolental fibroplasia
Abnormal vascularization at the back of the
eyes of preterm infants nursed in high oxygen
concentrations.

RLL
Right lobe of liver
See under RHL.
(see LHL, LLL)

RLL
Right lower lobe
Posteroinferior anatomical division of the
right lung.
(see CXR, LLL, LUL, RML, RUL)

RLPV
Right lower pulmonary vein
Vein draining the right lower lobe of
the lung.

RLQ

Right lower quadrant
Non-anatomical term used to describe right
inferior quarter of the abdomen (or breast).
LRQ

RLR

Right lateral rectus
Extra-ocular muscle abducting the right eye.

R–L shunt

Right to left shunt
Pathological connection between the
pulmonary and systemic circulation such that
blood bypasses the lungs and is not
oxygenated. Patient is often cyanosed.

RLZ

Right lower zone
Lower third of right lung field on a frontal
chest radiograph, below 4th anterior rib.
(see CXR, RLL, RMZ, RUZ)

RM

Radical mastectomy
Surgical removal of breast, underlying muscle
and axillary lymph nodes on the side affected
by carcinoma of the breast.

RM

Range of movement
Usually referring to joints.
ROM

RMA

Right mento anterior
Position of fetus in utero.

RMB

**Right mainstem bronchus / right main
bronchus**
See under RB.

RMBF

Regional myocardial blood flow
The relative perfusion of different cardiac
regions. Areas of cardiac ischaemia and
infarction can be distinguished by radionuclide
imaging.

RMCA

Right middle cerebral artery
Main terminal branch of the right internal
carotid artery supplying temporal and parietal
cerebral lobes.

RML

Right mediolateral
Site of episiotomy incision in perineum.

RML

Right middle lobe
Central anterior anatomical division of the
right lung.
ML
(see CXR, RLL, RUL)

RMO

Resident medical officer
Duty doctor in hospital, usually responsible for
management of admissions.

RMP

Regional myocardial perfusion
See under RMBF.

RMP

Right mento posterior
Position of fetus in utero.

RMR

Right medial rectus
Extra-ocular muscle adducting the right eye.

RMSF

Rocky mountain spotted fever
Tick-borne rickettsial illness endemic to
North and South America with clinical
features similar to epidemic typhus.

RMT

Right mento transverse
Position of fetus in utero.

RMV

Respiratory minute volume
Total amount of air moved into the lungs and
airways every minute, equal to the product of
the tidal volume and respiratory rate.

RMZ

Right mid-zone
Mid-third of the right lung field on a frontal
chest radiograph, between 2nd and 4th
anterior ribs.
(see CXR, RML, RLZ, RUZ)

RNA

Radionuclide angiography
Imaging of major blood vessels using
radiolabelled red blood cells.

RNA

Ribonucleic acid
Nucleic acid which transcribes information
from deoxyribonucleic acid (DNA) and acts as
a template for protein synthesis.
(see DNA)

RND
Radionuclide dacryocystography
Imaging of the tear duct using a radionuclide technique.

RNP
Ribonucleoprotein
Nuclear ribonucleoprotein antigen, characterizing 'mixed connective tissue disease' (MCTD), when antibodies are raised against it.
(*see anti-RNP*)

R/O
Rule out
Exclude.
TRO

ROC
Receiver operating characteristic
Study method to measure diagnostic performance (which is represented by the area under a curve drawn from the data).
ROC analysis

ROC analysis
Receiver operating characteristic analysis
See under ROC.

ROC curve
Receiver operating characteristic curve
Plot of the data obtained in a ROC study. Area under the resultant curve represents diagnostic performance.
(*see ROC*)

RöFo
Fortschritte auf dem Gebiet der Röntgenstrahlen
Official journal of the German and Austrian Röntgen Societies.

ROI
Region of interest
A selected area initially outlined on a soft copy image using a software drawing tool.

ROM
Range of movement
See under RM.

ROM
Read only memory
Area of the computer system from which information can be read but not changed.

ROM
Reduction of movement
Usually referring to joints.

ROM
Removal of metal
Removal of fixation pins or plates in orthopaedic surgery.

ROM
Rupture of membranes
The spontaneous or artificial breaking of the amniotic membranes surrounding the fetus, prior to delivery.
(*see ARM, AROM, IOL, SROM*)

ROP
Removal of pins
Removal of fixation pins in orthopaedic surgery.

ROP
Removal of plaster
Removal of plaster of Paris.

ROPE
Respiratory-ordered phase encoding
Process of varying the strength of phase encoding gradients in a non-sequential sequence in magnetic resonance imaging. Diminishes respiratory motion artefacts.

ROS
Review of systems / symptoms
Checklist of questions used in medical history taking to ensure no obvious symptoms are overlooked.
FE, SCL, SE, SR

RP
Retinitis pigmentosa
Triad of night blindness, peripheral visual field constriction, and a pigmentary retinopathy. Due to a metabolic disturbance in the outer retina. 50% are hereditary. May be associated with rare systemic syndromes.

RPA
Radiation protection adviser
Suitably qualified and experienced physicist advising District Health Authorities on matters relating to radiation protection.

RPA
Right pulmonary artery
Right terminal division of main pulmonary artery supplying the right lung.

RPGN
Rapidly progressive glomerulonephritis
Type of renal parenchymal disease leading to chronic renal failure.
(*see CGN, CRF, GN*)

RPE
Retinal pigment epithelium
Layer of phagocytic cells forming part of the outer retina of the eye where photochemical changes related to visual stimuli occur.

rpm
Revolutions per minute
Number of turns occurring in a minute.

RPO
Right posterior oblique
Radiographic projection in which the right posterior oblique part of the patient is nearest to the cassette, film or image-intensifier (IT).

RPP
Retropubic prostatectomy
Operative removal of the prostate gland via an abdominal incision.

RPRF
Rapidly progressive renal failure
A rapid deterioration in kidney function (occurring in days or weeks) resulting in the inadequate elimination of toxic metabolic products.
(see ATN, CRF, RF)

RPS
Radiation protection supervisor
Competent full-time employee in each department in which radiation is used who ensures all agreed protective measures are implemented.

RPT
Renal parenchymal thickness
Measurement of the width of kidney tissue (usually made ultrasonographically).

RPV
Right portal vein
Right branch of the hepatic portal vein.
(see HPV, MPV, PV)

RQ
Respiratory quotient
The ratio of the volume of carbon dioxide produced in respiration to the volume of oxygen used. The values indicate the type of food being metabolized.

R&R
Rate and rhythm
Speed and regularity of arterial pulsation.

R&R
Rest and relaxation
Allocates leisure time.

RR
Recovery room
Ward for patient care immediately following an interventional procedure, an operation or anaesthesia.

RR
Respiratory rate
Number of breaths per minute.

Rr
Rami
Branches, e.g. of nerves.

RS
Respiratory system
Upper airways, trachea, bronchial tree and lungs.

RS
Right septal
Pertaining to one of the internal heart walls as seen on echocardiography.

RSA
Right sacro anterior
Position of fetus in utero.

RSC
Right subclavian
Usually in respect of the position of an intravenous line.

RscA
Right scapulo anterior
Position of fetus in utero.

RSD
Reflex sympathetic dystrophy
Soft tissue and bony changes of unknown origin mediated by the sympathetic nervous system. Sudeck's atrophy.
RSDS

RSDS
Reflex sympathtic dystrophy syndrome
See under RSD.

RSIVP
Rapid sequence intravenous pyelogram
Contrast imaging of renal tract tailored to demonstrate renal ischaemia if present. Films are taken 1, 2, 3, 5 and 10 minutes after a rapid injection of contrast medium. Now obsolete.

RSL
Right sacro lateral
Position of fetus *in utero*.

RSM
Royal Society of Medicine
British medical society open to all medical practitioners.

RSNA
The Radiological Society of North America
1. Official US American radiological body.
2. The annual conference of the Radiological Society of North America, which is currently the largest and most important international radiological meeting.
(see EAR, ECR)

RSO
Resident Surgical Officer
Senior resident surgeon in a hospital.

RSU
Radiological Sciences Unit
Department of imaging encompassing related disciplines such as medical physics.

RSV
Respiratory syncytial virus
Ribonucleic acid (RNA) paramyxovirus. Important cause of respiratory infection in infants and small children.

RT
Radiotherapy
Treatment of neoplastic disease using high voltage radiation.
DXR, DXT

RT
Rectal temperature

Rt
Right
(see Lt)

RTA
Renal tubular acidosis
Inability of the kidney to excrete acid urine resulting in a systemic metabolic acidosis.

RTA
Road traffic accident
MVA

RTD
Renal tubule/tubular defects
Syndrome encompassing a large number of acquired or hereditary disorders affecting tubules rather than glomeruli.

RTFM
Read the manual
An impolite suggestion that the instructions booklet should be consulted.
RTM

RTM
Read the manual
A suggestion that the instructions booklet should be consulted.
(see RTFM)

rTPA/rtPA
Recombinant tissue plasminogen activator
Genetically synthesized thrombolytic agent used in treatment of myocardial infarction and peripheral blood clot.
(see TPA/tPA)

RTU
Renal transplant unit
Hospital ward which cares for patients who have undergone kidney transplantation.

RUA
Reduction under anaesthesia
External manipulation of a fracture requiring general anaesthesia.
(see EUA, MUA)

RU
Right upper extremity
Right arm or hand.

RUL
Right upper lobe
Anatomical division of right lung.
(see CXR, RLL, RML, LLL, LUL)

RUO
Right ureteric orifice
Opening of the right ureter into the bladder.

RUOQ
Right upper outer quadrant
Right supero-lateral quarter (of the breast).

RUPV
Right upper pulmonary vein
Blood vessel draining upper lobe of the right lung.

RUQ
Right upper quadrant
Non-anatomical term used to describe right superior quarter of the abdomen (or breast).

RUZ
Right upper zone
Upper third of the right lung field on a frontal chest radiograph, above the 2nd anterior rib.
(see CXR, RLZ, RMZ, RUL)

RV
Residual volume
Volume of air remaining in lungs following a maximal expiration.
(see FEV, IC, IRC, TLC)

RV
Right ventricle
Right heart chamber pumping blood to pulmonary circulation.
(see LV)

RV
Right ventricular branch
Branch of the right coronary artery.

RVEF
Right ventricular ejection fraction
Amount of blood, expressed as a percentage of the end-diastolic right ventricular volume, ejected from the right ventricle during one cardiac cycle.
(see EF, LVEF)

RVF
Right ventricular failure
See under RHF.
(see CCF, HF, LHF, LVF)

RVH
Right ventricular hypertrophy
Increased muscular mass of the right cardiac ventricle.
(see LVH)

RVOT
Right ventricular outflow tract
Course taken by blood ejected from the right ventricle past the pulmonary valve into the pulmonary artery.
(see LVOT)

RVT
Renal vein thrombosis
Blood clot in the renal vein, associated with nephrotic syndrome and glomerulonephritis.

RVV
Right ventricular volume
Volume of blood in the right ventricle at the end of diastole.
TRVV

RVWT
Right ventricular wall thickness
Width of the muscle of the right cardiac ventricle.

Rx
Therapy / treatment
Corrupted abbreviation for 'recipe'. Latin for 'take thou'. Used as an instruction on written prescriptions.

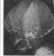

Σ
Syphilis
A sexually and congenitally transmitted disease, with chronic multisystem manifestations, caused by the spirochaete *Treponema pallidum*.

1st S
First septal perforator
Branch of left anterior descending coronary artery.

s
Second
SI unit of time (t).
(see min, h, t)

s
Specific heat capacity
The heat required to raise unit mass of a substance by unit temperature.

S
Septal perforating arteries
Branches of the left anterior descending coronary artery supplying the interventricular septum.

S
Sigmoid colon
S-shaped pelvic portion of the large bowel between the rectum and descending colon.
Σ, SC

S
Sigmoidoscopy
Examination of the distal large bowel with a rigid or flexible endoscope.

S_1
First heart sound
Caused by closure of mitral and tricuspid valves.

S_2
Second heart sound
Caused by closure of aortic and pulmonary valves.

SA
Surface area

SA
System administrator
Person who runs a host computer system or public access site.
Sysadmin.

SACE
Serum angiotensin converting enzyme
Blood level of enzyme responsible for production of Angiotensin 2, a powerful endogenous vasoconstrictor. Raised in sarcoidosis.

SAD
Seasonal affective disorder
Syndrome of depression occurring during the winter months.

SAE
Subcortical arteriosclerotic encephalopathy
Hypertension-induced vascular ischaemic damage in the periventricular white matter. Binswanger disease.

sag.
Sagittal (Latin: *Sagitta*. Literally 'an arrow')
Body plane passing anterior to posterior in longitudinal section, i.e. in a plane parallel to the sagittal suture of the skull.

SAH
Subarachnoid haemorrhage
Bleeding into the subarachnoid space of the meninges. Commonly follows rupture of an aneurysm or arteriovenous malformation.

Salp.
Salpingectomy
Surgical removal of a Fallopian tube.
Salpx.
(see BSO)

Salp.
Salpingography
Radiocontrast investigation of the Fallopian tube(s).
(see HSG)

SALP
Serum alkaline phosphatase
Enzyme present in liver, bone and placenta. A raised serum levels indicates either liver or bone disease, or pregnancy.
alk. phos., ALP

Salpx.
Salpingectomy
See under Salp.
(see BSO)

SAM

Self-administered morphine
Intravenous bolus infusion of morphine
analgesia controlled by patient so that the dose
can be suited to the level of pain.
(see PCA)

SAM

Systolic anterior motion of mitral valve
Characteristic finding on echocardiography in
hypertrophic obstructive cardiomyopathy
(HOCM).

SAN

Sinu-atrial node
The natural 'pacemaker' of the heart which
initiates each cardiac cycle.

SAP

Serum amyloid protein
Component of amyloid used as a tracer when
labelled with iodine-123 for the detection of
systemic amyloid.

SAP

Systolic arterial pressure
Systemic arterial blood pressure during
ventricular contraction.

SAPF

Simultaneous anterior and posterior fusion
Surgical procedure for stabilizing the spine
using bone grafts.

SAR

Specific absorption rate
Rate at which energy is deposited in magnetic
resonance imaging, usually in W kg^{-1}.

SARA

Sexually acquired reactive arthritis
Joint disease associated with a sexually
transmitted disease (SDT).
(see VD)

SAS

Subaortic stenosis
Narrowing of the left ventricular outflow tract
below the aortic valve.

SAT

Systolic acceleration time
Duration of systolic up-stroke of flow in a
vessel investigated by spectral Doppler
ultrasound (US).

SATL

Surgical Achilles tendon lengthening
Operation to stretch the main ankle tendon.

S. aureus

Staphylococcus aureus
Gram-positive bacterium; a common cause of
cutaneous infection, arthritis, osteomyelitis,
and endocarditis.

Sax

Short axis
The smallest cross-sectional dimension.
E.g. may refer to a specific orientation of an
echocardiography ultrasound probe, or to a
lymph node dimension.

SB

Stillbirth
Baby born dead after at least 28 weeks'
gestation.

SBE

Small bowel enema
Contrast examination of jejunum and ileum
obtained by cannulating the terminal
duodenum (*per oram*) and instilling dilute
barium. Enteroclysis.

SBE

Subacute bacterial endocarditis
Infection of the endothelial lining of the heart,
commonly in association with
an abnormal or prosthetic heart valve in the
presence of a bacteraemia.
(see ABE, BE, IE)

SBO

Small bowel obstruction
Blockage in the small bowel that may be
intrinsic, extrinsic or metabolic in origin.

SBP

Spontaneous bacterial peritonitis
Infection of ascitic fluid, commonly following
bacteraemia in a cirrhotic patient.

SBP

Systolic blood pressure
Highest point of systemic arterial blood
pressure in the cardiac cycle.
SP

SC

Sclerosing cholangitis
Hepatobiliary disorder characterized by
progressive biliary fibrosis and, ultimately,
biliary cirrhosis and hepatocellular failure.
PSC

SC

Sigmoid colon
See under S.

SC, S/C
Subcutaneous
Under the skin. A common site for injections.
Sub. cut.

S/C
Sugar-coated
Tablet with an outer layer of a sugary
substance.

SCA
Sickle cell anaemia
Haemolytic anaemia caused by the
homozygous inheritance of a gene causing the
synthesis of abnormal haemoglobin (Hb S).
This causes the red blood cells to assume a
crescent shape under stress.
SCD

SCA+
Sheep cell agglutination test
An assay of the concentration of specific
antibodies present. The degree of clumping
they cause in antigen-coated sheep red blood
cells is measured.

SCAR
**Society for Computer Applications in
Radiology**
Organization based in the States concerned
with computer and communication
technologies applied to radiology and digital
imaging.

SCB
Strictly confined to bed
Patient not allowed out of bed for any purpose.
ABR

SCBE
Single contrast barium enema
Imaging of colon using barium alone.
(see BE, DCBE)

SCBU
Special care baby unit
Ward for premature and sick newborn babies.
NICU, NNU

SCC
Squamous cell carcinoma
Malignant epithelial tumour.
(see BCC)

SCCL
Small cell carcinoma of lung
Radiosensitive malignant tumour composed of
small, oval, undifferentiated cells: 'oat cell
carcinoma'.

SCD
Scleroderma
Multisystem disorder characterized by fibrosis
of the skin, blood vessels and visceral organs,
such as gastrointestinal tract, lungs and
kidneys. Often associated with CREST
syndrome.
PSS, SS

SCD
Sickle cell disease
See under SCA.

SCD
Sudden cardiac death
Death within hours or minutes of the
onset of ischaemic cardiac pain or without
warning.
SHD
(see SUD)

ScDA
Scapulo dextra anterior
Position of fetus in utero.

ScDP
Scapulo dextra posterior
Position of fetus in utero.

SCID
Soft copy image display
Demonstration of digital images on monitors.

SCL
Symptom check list
Systematic review of symptoms which may not
have been volunteered by a patient.
FE, ROS, SE, SR

ScLA
Scapulo laeva anterior
Position of fetus in utero.

SCLC
Squamous cell lung carcinoma
Type of lung cancer, as determined by
histology or cytology.

ScLP
Scapulo laeva posterior
Position of fetus in utero.

SCM
Sternocleidomastoid
Neck muscle supplied by the accessory nerve
(CNXI). Turns the head and is an accessory
muscle of respiration.

SCP

Service class provider
The device (e.g. an archive) acting as a
'server' in a DICOM standard network
(e.g. by receiving images).

SCRF

Surface coil rotating frame
Magnetic resonance spectroscopy technique
using surface coils taking advantage of spins
near the surface.
RFS

SCU

Service class user
The device (e.g. a scanner) acting as a 'client'
in a DICOM standard network (e.g. by
sending images).

SCVIR

**Society of Cardiovascular and Interventional
Radiology**
American society concerned with the practice
and teaching of cardiovascular and
interventional radiology.
(see APSCVIR, BSIR, CIRSE, JSAIR, JVIR,
WAIS)

SCWM

Subcortical white matter
That area of 'conducting' myelinated neurones
which underlies the cerebral cortex.

SD

Senile dementia
Worsening of memory and intellectual
deterioration without impairment of
consciousness in the elderly.

SD

Septal defect
'Hole in the heart', either between the
ventricles or the atria, allowing abnormal
shunting of the blood.

SD

Skin dose
Amount of energy imparted to the skin by
radiation incident upon it.

SD

Spontaneous delivery
Normal childbirth.
NVD, SVD

SD

Standard deviation
Statistical term for describing the spread of a
Gaussian curve in a population or a range of
values around the mean expected from random
variation.

SDH

Sub-dural haemorrhage
Bleeding into the sub-dural space of the
meninges.

SDMS

Society of Diagnostic Medical Sonographers
Professional organization of ultrasonographers;
publishes the *Journal of Diagnostic Medical
Sonography*.

SDP

Sacro dextra posterior
Fetal position, with the sacrum towards the
right and the back.

SDS

Shy-Drager syndrome
Neurodegenerative disease characterized
clinically by autonomic nervous system failure.

SDSL

Symmetrical digital single line
Means of sending digital images: a
bidirectional line.

SDT

Sacro dextra transversa
Fetal position, with the sacrum to the right
side.

SE

Side effect
Unwanted effect of a drug or treatment.

SE

Spin echo
Sequence of radiofrequency pulses in magnetic
resonance imaging whereby the signal
reappears after reversal of the dephasing
proton spins.

SE

Systematic enquiry
See under SCL.
FE, ROS, SR

Se

Selenium
Main constituent of a xeroradiography plate.
Acts as a semiconductor.
(see Al, Al$_2$O$_3$)

^{75}Se, 75-Se

Selenium-75
Radionuclide used in nuclear medicine for investigation of bile malabsorption and for localization of adrenal tumours.

sec

Second
See under s.
(see h, min, t)

SECAM

Séquence à mémoire
Defines video connection standard used in France. Means of encoding colour information on a television signal.

SeHCAT

Se^{75} haemofolic acid taurine
Radioisotope tracer used to investigate malabsorption of bile acids.

SEM

Scanning electron microscope
Instrument for three-dimensional imaging of objects too small to be resolved by light beams. Images are formed using electrons reflected from a specially prepared specimen.

SEM

Standard error of the mean
Term used in medical statistics. Range of error likely to occur when estimating the mean value within a sample.

SEM

Systolic ejection murmur
Turbulent blood flow audible on auscultation, synchronous with ventricular contraction (carotid pulsation). The intensity rises then falls, being loudest in mid-systole.
ESM

SEMI

Subendocardial myocardial infarction
Single or multiple foci of necrosis in the inner ventricular wall resulting from atherosclerotic coronary artery stenosis.
(see MI)

SEN

State-enrolled nurse
Qualified nurse who has undergone two years of predominantly practical training.

SER

Somatosensory evoked responses
Study of electrical activity at any point in the sensory pathway in response to small painless electrical stimuli which are administered to the large sensory nerves in the hand or leg.

SES

Spheno ethmoidal suture
Joint between the ethmoid and sphenoid bones in the skull.

SF

Screen-film
Conventional X-ray film used with an intensifying screen.
(see IP, PPP, PSP)

SFA

Superficial femoral artery
Main branch of the femoral artery which becomes the popliteal artery at the adductor canal above the knee.

SFD

Small for dates
Fetus smaller than expected from the time spent in utero.
SGA

SFE

Slipped femoral epiphysis
Displacement downwards and backwards of the epiphysis of the femoral head. Causes painful hip(s) in children aged 10 to 16, commoner in boys.
SUFE

SFJ

Saphenofemoral junction
Link between the long saphenous and femoral veins, i.e. between the superficial and deep lower limb venous systems.

SFS

Shared file server
Central disc shared by a number of computers.

SFS

Spatial freqency spectrum
Distribution of the spatial frequencies of an object as expressed by a Fourier analysis.

SG

Specific gravity
The ratio of the density of a substance to that of water.
Sp. Gr.

SGA
Small for gestational age
See under SFD.

SGOT
Serum glutamic oxaloacetic transaminase
Enzyme present in the liver and heart. A raised serum level indicates disease of either of these organs. Aspartate transaminase is the new name for this enzyme.
AST

SGPT
Serum glutamic pyruvic transaminase
Hepatocellular enzyme. Elevated serum levels indicate liver disease.
ALT

SH
Social history
Details of patient's employment, marital status, hobbies, alcohol, drug and tobacco intake and housing.

SH
Surgical history
Details of patient's previous operations and anaesthetics.
PSH

Sh
Shigella
Group of gram-negative bacteria that cause intestinal infection.

SHBG
Sex hormone binding globulin
A blood protein which binds testosterone as an inactive complex.

SHD
Sudden heart death
See under SCD.
(*see SUD*)

SHO
Senior House Officer
Post-registration junior hospital doctor.
(*see HP, HS*)

sHPT
Secondary hyperparathyroidism
Raised serum parathyroid hormone to compensate for a low serum calcium, such as may occur in renal disease.
$2°$ HPT

SI
Signal intensity
Strength of the signal from a voxel of tissue as detected by a magnetic resonance scanner (MRI scanner).

sic
Latin: so or thus
Textual annotation, usually inserted in brackets to indicate that an odd or questionable allusion is in fact accurate.

SII
Self-inflicted injury
Deliberately perpetrated self harm, e.g. to obtain attention or hospital admission.

SI joint
Sacro iliac joint
Joint between the sacrum and the iliac bone. Largest joint in the body.
SIJ

si op sit
si opus sit
From the Latin: 'if there is need'. If necessary.
SOS

SI unit
Système International d'Unités
International system of units recommended for all scientific purposes.

si vir perm
Si vires permittant
If strength permits.

SIADH
Syndrome of inappropriate anti-diuretic hormone secretion
Clinical entity of diverse aetiology, characterized by an inappropriate oversecretion of anti-diuretic hormone (ADH) causing water retention.

sid
Semel in die
Once daily.
od

SIDS
Sudden infant death syndrome
Unexplained death in infants aged 1 month to 1 year without readily identifiable cause. 'Cot death'.
SUDI

SIJ
Sacro iliac joint
See under SI joint.

SIMV

Synchronized intermittent mandatory ventilation
Artificial ventilation involving the periodic delivery of breaths synchronized with, and additional to spontaneous patient breathing.

sin.

sine
Periodic mathematical function. Ratio of opposite / hypotenuse sides of a triangle.

SIN

Salpingitis isthmica nodosa
Ectatic abnormality of the Fallopian tubes usually following genitourinary infection.

SIW

Self-inflicted wound
Deliberately self-perpetrated injury, e.g. to seek attention or hospital admission.
(see DSH, SII)

SK

Streptokinase
Thrombolytic agent used in treatment of myocardial infarction.

SL, S/L

Sublingual
Under the tongue. Route of drug administration for absorption via buccal mucosa. Site of temperature measurement.

SLA

Sacro leva anterior
Position of fetus in utero, with the sacrum to the left and to the front.

SLE

Systemic lupus erythematosus
Multi-system vasculitis of unknown aetiology which is probably immunologically mediated. An important cause of renal disease.
DLE, LE

SLIP

Serial line Internet protocol
Means whereby home computers are turned into Internet sites over a telephone line.

SLP

Sacro leva posterior
Position of fetus in utero, with the sacrum to the left and to the back.

SLS

Stein–Leventhal syndrome
Obesity, hirsutism, virilism and irregular menses in association with enlarged polycystic ovaries.

SLT

Sacro laeva transversa
Position of fetus in utero, with the sacrum to the left.

SM

Sado-masochism
Deviant sexual behaviour associated with the infliction of pain and unusual trauma.
(see B&D)

SM

Simple mastectomy
Surgical removal of the breast without removal of muscle or axillary nodes.

SM

Systolic murmur
Turbulent flow, audible on auscultation during ventricular contraction.
(see ESM)

SMA

Anti-smooth muscle antibody
Antibody used as a marker for autoimmune disease of the liver, especially chronic active hepatitis (CAH).

SMA

Spinal muscular atrophy
Variety of motor neurone disease in which peripheral motor neurones are affected without evidence of involvement of the corticospinal system.

SMA

Superior mesenteric artery
Main visceral vessel supplying pancreas, small intestine and colon proximal to the splenic flexure, i.e. the entire primitive mid-gut.

SMI

Silent myocardial infarction
Asymptomatic irreversible necrosis of heart muscle.

Smith's

Smith's fracture
Fracture of the distal radius with volar angulation.
(see Colles')

SMPTE
Society of Motion Picture and Television Engineers
Body which defined a test pattern widely used for image quality.

SMR
Standardized mortality ratio
Ratio of mortality rates in a given socioeconomic group compared with that of the general population.

SMR
Submucous resection
Plastic surgery to bone and cartilage of nasal septum.

SMV
Superior mesenteric vein
Portal venous tributary draining pancreas, small bowel and colon proximal to splenic flexure.

SN
Sinus node artery
Branch of right coronary artery.

S/N
Signal to noise ratio
Ratio of signal from an imaged object to random signal fluctuations as recorded by an imaging system. The higher the SNR, the better the image contrast.
SNR

SNDO
Standard nomenclature of diseases and operations
A classification system.

SNF
Skilled nursing facility
Ward providing intensive nursing care.
HDU

SNIPA
Seronegative inflammatory polyarthritis
Inflammatory joint disease in which rheumatoid factor is absent from the serum.

SNM
Society of Nuclear Medicine
American body of nuclear medicine physicians.

SNMT
Society of Nuclear Medicine Technicians
American body of nuclear medicine technicians.

SNR
Signal to noise ratio
See under S/N.

SNS
Sympathetic nervous system
Part of the nervous system controlling the visceral functions of the body. Uses noradrenaline as the neurotransmitter in post-ganglionic neurones. Responsible for 'fight or flight' reactions.

SNSA
Seronegative spondyloarthropathy
HLA B 27-associated inflammatory bone and joint disease.

SO
Salpingo-oophorectomy
Surgical removal of ovary and ipsilateral Fallopian tube.

SO
Superior oblique
Ocular muscle innervated by the fourth cranial nerve (CNIV). Moves eye downwards and outwards.

SOAP
Subjective, objective, assessment/plan
Formal method for recording patient progress.

SOB
Shortness of breath
DIB, dysp.
(*see* DOE, SOBOE)

SOBOE
Shortness of breath on exertion
DOE
(*see* DIB, SOB)

SOC
Synovial osteochondromatosis
A benign disease of joint synovium involving inflammation, proliferation and metaplasia.

SOD
Superoxide dismutase
An enzyme which quenches superoxide ions thus protecting cells from oxygen toxicity.

SOL
Space occupying lesion
Any discrete pathological entity which exerts mass effect. Includes tumour, abscess, aneurysm, haematoma, granuloma and cyst.

SOM
Secretory otitis media
Middle ear infection with discharge.

SONET
Synchronous optical network
A standard for using optical media to interconnect high-speed networks.

SONH
Spontaneous osteonecrosis of the hip
Avascular necrosis (AVN) of the hip caused by a variety of medical and surgical conditions such as trauma, vasculitis, blood disorders or steroid medication.
(see ON, SONK)

SONK
Spontaneous osteonecrosis of the knee
Avascular necrosis (AVN) of the knee usually involving the medial condyle of the femur.
(see ON, SONH)

SOP
Service object pair
A DICOM standard definition which describes both the information object to be transferred (e.g. a digital medical image) and the command to be performed (e.g. storing that image).

SOPI
Service object pair instance
A specific service object pair (SOP).

SOREM
Sleep onset rapid eye movement
Deep sleep associated with rapid eye movement, during which dreaming occurs.
REM

SOS
Save our souls
Plea for emergency assistance.

SOS
Si opus sit
See under si op sit.

SOW
System of work
Written procedures designed to ensure that staff entering a radiation controlled area do not exceed ⅒ of any annual dose limit.

S/P
Status post
Condition of a patient following a clinical event, e.g. an operation.

SP
Suprapubic
Above symphysis pubis, may refer to disease location or to operative or interventional access route.

SP
Systolic pressure
See under SBP.

Sp. Cd
Spinal cord

Sp. fl.
Spinal fluid
Fluid bathing the brain and spinal cord.
CSF

Sp. Gr.
Specific gravity
See under SG.

SPIE
Society of Photo-optical Instrument Engineers
Organization based in the USA concerned with computer and communication technologies applied to digital imaging in medical diagnosis and therapy.

Sp.
Species
Form of, type of.

Sp.
Specimen
Sample taken for diagnostic examination or evaluation.

Sp.
Special
Particular, set apart from, distinguished.

Sp.
Specific
Explicit, particular, definite.

Sp. Pn.
Spontaneous pneumothorax
Escape of air into the pleural space without predisposing underlying lung disorder or other precipitating factor.
Sp. Pnx

Sp. Pnx
Spontaneous pneumothorax
See under Sp. Pn.

SPACE

Single potential analysis of cavernous electrical activity
Investigation of the autonomic nervous supply of the penis.

SPAF

Spontaneous paroxysmal atrial fibrillation
Sudden onset of continuous rapid electrical activation of the atria with little/no mechanical activity and irregular conduction to the ventricles.

SPECT

Single photon emission computed tomography
Planar method of image acquisition in nuclear medicine enabling 3-D image reconstruction.
ECT

SPG

Splenoportography
Contrast examination of the splenic and hepatic portal veins using an injection into the splenic pulp.

SPGR

Spoiled gradient-refocused acquisition in the steady state (GRASS)
Heavily T1-weighted radiofrequency spoiled gradient echo technique in General Electric machines.

SPI

Standard product interconnect
An extension to the ACR-NEMA standard whereby each digital image is uniquely identified in the global context by its country, manufacturer and system code.

SPIH

Superimposed pregnancy induced hypertension
High blood pressure developing in pregnancy.

Spiral CT

Spiral computed tomography
Form of computed tomography (CT) acquiring three dimensional (3D) data set with continuously rotating X-ray tube and moving patient table.
Helical CT

SPJ

Saphenopopliteal junction
Link between the short saphenous and popliteal veins connecting the superficial and deep lower limb venous systems.

S. pyogenes

Streptococcus pyogenes
Streptococcal Group A bacterium; commonly causing acute pyogenic (pus forming) infections, rheumatic fever and glomerulonephritis.

SQL

Structured query language
Allows data to be retrieved from (and inserted into) a database using its attributes to search the relational database table.

SR

Saturation recovery
Pulse sequence in magnetic resonance imaging characterized by two sequential 90-degree pulses; a saturation and a detection pulse. This results in short repetition time spin echo (SE) sequences.

SR

Senior registrar (US: Senior Resident)
Highest grade of junior doctor, i.e. highest training grade.

SR

Sinus rhythm
Normal cardiac electrical cycle, initiated by the sinu-atrial node (SAN).

SR

Slow release
Drug preparation which dissolves slowly.

SR

Systems review
Checklist of questions used in medical history taking to ensure no obvious symptoms are overlooked.
FE, ROS, SE

85Sr, Sr-85

Strontium-85
Calcium analogue radionuclide formerly used in nuclear medicine for bone scanning. Has been replaced by technetium-99m (^{99m}Tc) methylene diphosphonate (MDP).
(*see* ^{87m}Sr)

87mSr, Sr-87m

Strontium-87m
Radionuclide formerly used in nuclear medicine for bone scanning. Has been replaced by technetium-99m (^{99m}Tc) methylene diphosphonate (MDP).
(*see* ^{85}Sr)

SRN
State registered nurse
Former term for registered general nurse (RGN).

SROM
Spontaneous rupture of membranes
The spontaneous breaking of the amniotic membranes surrounding the fetus, prior to delivery.
(see ARM, AROM, IOL, ROM)

SRSA
Slow reacting substance of anaphylaxis
Immunological agent causing prolonged smooth muscle contraction in allergic reactions.

SS
Sjögren's syndrome
Immunological disorder characterized by exocrine gland destruction, causing mucosal and conjunctival dryness, and a variety of autoimmune phenomena.

SS
Systemic sclerosis
See under SCD.
PSS
(see CREST)

SSCT
Stereotactic subcaudate tractotomy
Pyschosurgical management of resistant affective and compulsive disorders.

SSD
Shaded surface display
A reconstruction algorithm used to generate three dimensional (3D) computed tomography (CT) images.
(see MIP, VRT)

SSFP
Steady state free precession
Method of magnetic resonance excitation in which radiofrequency pulses are applied rapidly and repeatedly.

SSM
Superficial spreading melanoma
Skin malignancy. Radial growth predominates for months or years before invasion occurs.

SSP
Section sensitivity profile
Dimensions and characteristics of a voxel along the longitudinal axis (Z Line).

SSPE
Subacute sclerosing panencephalitis
Progressive inflammation of cerebral substance occurring several years after measles infection.

SSRI
Selective serotonin reuptake inhibitor
Antidepressant drug with specific activity on synapses involving the neurotransmitter serotonin.

SSS
Sick sinus syndrome
Cardiac conduction defect of the sinu-atrial node, causing brady/tachy-arrhythmias.
(see BTS)

SSS
Superior sagittal sinus
Large dural sinus of the brain which lies in the interhemispheric fissure and drains into the torcula herophili.

SSSS
Staphylococcal scalded skin syndrome
Generalized exfoliative dermatitis complicating infection by toxin-producing strains of Staphylococcus aureus.

ST segment
Part of the electrocardiographic (ECG) trace between the S and T waves which may be altered in pathological states (e.g. angina, hypertension, cardiomyopathy).

STANDOUT
Soft thresholding and depth cueing of unspecified techniques
Post-processing technique used for three dimensional (3D) reconstructions in magnetic resonance imaging (MRI).

Staph.
Staphylococcus / staphlococci
Common bacterial pathogens. The various species cause skin and wound infections as well as pneumonia, osteomyelitis and endocarditis.

Stat.
Statim
Immediately; as initial dose.

Stb
Stillborn
Baby born dead after at least 28 weeks gestation.

STD

Sexually transmitted disease
Diseases contracted principally through sexual contact.
VD

STEAM

Stimulated-echo acquisition mode
Magnetic resonance fast-imaging technique using two 90-degree radiofrequency pulses followed by a third pulse of 90 degrees or less. Subsequent spin echoes are produced as 'stimulated echoes'.

STEN

Staphylococcal toxic epidermal necrolysis
Epidermal cell death in response to staphylococcal toxins or drug reaction. May be lethal.
TEN

STIR

Short tau inversion recovery
Magnetic resonance sequence used to suppress the signal returned from fatty tissues.
(*see Fat. Sat.*)

STM

Short term memory
Ability to recall recent events.

STOP

Surgical termination of pregnancy
Surgical abortion.
TAB, TOP

STP

Shielded twisted pair
Insulated cable pairs covered by shielding conductor. Gives good noise protection.

STP

Standard temperature and pressure
Standard conditions used as basis for calculations involving quantities varying with temperature (T) and pressure (P). Defined as 273.15°Kelvin (K) and 101325 pascal (Pa).
NTP

Str.

Streptococcus / streptococci
Common bacterial pathogens causing a variety of diseases, particularly throat, wound and skin infections.

Strep.

Streptococcus / streptococci
See under Str.

Sub. cut.

Subcutaneous
See under SC.

SUD

Sudden unexpected death
Death without previous symptoms, invariably due to cardiac or vascular collapse.
(*see SCD*)

SUDI

Sudden unexpected death in infancy
See under SIDS.

SUFE

Slipped upper femoral epiphysis
See under SFE.

sup.

Superior
Used in anatomical descriptions to denote a cephalad situation relative to a reference structure.
(*see ant., inf., post.*)

SV

Selective vagotomy
Surgical transection of each vagus nerve just beyond its bifurcation into gastric and extragastric divisions. Treatment for peptic ulcer, now largely obsolete.
(*see HSV*)

SV

Stroke volume
Volume of blood ejected from the heart during systole.

Sv

Sievert
Unit of dose equivalent (H) and effective dose equivalent (EDE). Takes into account the different radiobiological effectiveness (RBE) of various types of radiation. 1 Sv = 1 gray (Gy) quality factor (QF).
(*see mSv*)

SVA

Selective visceral angiography
Contrast imaging of intra-abdominal arterial branches by individual catheterization and opacification.

SVAS

Supravalvular aortic stenosis
Left ventricular outflow narrowing above aortic valve. Rarely, generalized hypoplasia of ascending aorta.

SVBG

Saphenous vein bypass graft
Surgical treatment of coronary arterial stenosis using a leg vein.
(*see* CABG)

SVC

Superior vena cava
Main vein draining the body above the heart.

SVCO

Superior vena cava obstruction
Obstruction of the superior vena cava causing distended neck veins, facial oedema and blackouts.
SVCS

SVCS

Superior vena cava syndrome
See under SVCO.

SVD

Single vessel disease
Coronary arterial stenosis affecting only one vessel.

SVD

Spontaneous vaginal delivery
Normal delivery of baby, via the vagina.
NVD, SD

SVE

Supraventricular extrasystole
Atrial beat not followed by ventricular contraction.

SVGA / Super VGA

Super video graphics adaptors
High resolution display card and associated monitor widely used on IBM compatible personal computers.
(*see* EGA)

SVI

Slow virus infection
Infection with viral agent with a long latent period, usually presenting clinically with neurological symptoms and signs.
(*see* CJD, JCD, JKD, KJD)

SVI

Stroke volume index
Cardiac output per beat expressed as a fraction of body surface area.

SVR

Systemic vascular resistance
Opposition to blood flow offered by the entire systemic vascular tree.
PVR, TPR, TPVR, TSVR, TVR

SVT

Supraventricular tachycardia
Abnormal focus of electrical activity in the atria or conducting system above the ventricles, causing rapid cardiac contractions.
(*see* PSVT)

S/W

Spike wave
Pattern of electrical complexes on an electroencephalogram. A frequency of 3 per second indicates petit mal epilepsy.

SWI

Stroke work index
The volume of blood ejected from the left ventricle in one contraction expressed as a fraction of body surface area.

Sx

Signs
Clinical abnormalities elicited on examination.

Sx

Symptoms
Patients' complaints about how they feel.

SXR

Skull X-ray

Syn.

Synonym
A word with the same or similar meaning to another.

Sysadmin.

System administrator
See under SA.

SYSOP

System operator
Person who runs a bulletin-board (on-line newsletter) on the Internet.

Syst.

Systemic
Throughout the body, e.g. widespread disease affecting multiple tissues, such as a vasculitis.

Syst.

Systolic
During cardiac ventricular contraction.

θ

Theta, tomograghic angle
Amplitude of tube travel in conventional tomography expressed in degrees. Slice thickness decreases with increasing θ and *vice versa*.

T$_{\frac{1}{2}}$

Half-life
Time after which radioactivity of a substance has decayed to half its original value.
(*see* T$_{\frac{1}{2}}$*biol,* T$_{\frac{1}{2}}$*eff,* T$_{\frac{1}{2}}$*phys*)

T$_1$

Longitudinal relaxation time
Time that it takes for longitudinal magnetization vector to recover in magnetic resonance imaging (MRI).
T1
(*see* T$_2$)

T1

Longitudinal relaxation time
See under T$_1$.
(*see* T$_2$)

T$_2$

Transverse relaxation time
Time that it takes for the transverse magnetization vector to recover in magnetic resonance imaging (MRI).
T2
(*see* T$_1$)

T2

Transverse relaxation time
See under T$_2$.
(*see* T$_1$)

T$_2$*

Effective transverse relaxation time
Refers to the situation in which the observed transverse relaxation time is faster than the normal T$_2$ time because of spatial inhomogeneity of the magnetic field.
T2*

T2*

Effective transverse relaxation time
See under T$_2$*.

T3

Tri-iodothyronine
Form of thyroxine. Elevated plasma levels of free tri-iodothyronine indicate hyperthyroidism.
(*see* T4)

T4

Thyroxine
Hormone produced by the thyroid which affects metabolism.
(*see* fT4, T3)

t

Time

T

Temperature

T

Tesla
SI unit of magnetic flux density.
(*see* G)

T

Thoracic nerve root
Used with a number 1–12 to define the root level.

T

Thoracic vertebra
Used with a number 1–12 to represent a particular vertebral level e.g. T10.
D (Dorsal)

T&A

Tonsillectomy and adenoidectomy
Surgical removal of tonsils and adenoids.

TA

Tibialis anterior
One of the arteries supplying the foot.

TA

Truncus arteriosus
Congenital cardiovascular anomaly in which a single large vessel receives all blood ejected from both sides of the heart.
Truncus
(*see* CHD)

TAA

Tumour associated antigen
Antigen present on tumour cells (but which may also occur on normal cells).

TAB

Therapeutic abortion
Surgical termination of pregnancy.
STOP, TOP

Tab.(s)

Tablet(s)
Pills.

Tab.

Tabulation
Margin indentation on a word processor or typewriter.

TAC

Time activity curve
Graph plotting radioactivity in a sample volume or region of interest (ROI) against time.

TAE

Transcatheter arterial embolization
Therapeutic occlusion of an artery by coils, particles or glue through an angiography catheter.

TAF

Tumor angiogenesis factor
Substance secreted by tumours which stimulates neovascularization.

TAH

Total abdominal hysterectomy
Surgical removal of uterus, via an abdominal incision.

TAHBSO

Total abdominal hysterectomy and bilateral salpingo-oophorectomy
Surgical removal of uterus, both Fallopian tubes and ovaries, via an abdominal incision.

TALL

T cell acute lymphoblastic leukaemia
Haematological malignancy caused by proliferation of immature T lymphocytes.

TAM

Time averaged mean
Average of the Doppler shift frequency of the signal from an artery over a cardiac cycle, used in the measurement of pulsatility index (PI).
TWA

TAMI

Transmural anterior myocardial infarction
Full thickness ischaemic death of cardiac tissue resulting from left anterior coronary artery occlusion.
(see AMI)

tan.

Tangent
Ratio of opposite/adjacent sides of a triangle.

TANSTAAFL

There ain't no such thing as a free lunch
You never get anything for nothing.

TAO

Thromboangiitis obliterans
Nervous and vascular inflammation, with thrombosis of small and medium-sized arteries, usually seen in young male smokers.

TAP

Transluminal angioplasty
Balloon dilatation of a vascular stenosis using a catheter inserted through the skin at a site distant from the stenosis.
PTA, TLA

TAPE

Temporary atrial pacemaker electrode
Device inserted into the atrium which supplies electrical stimulation to the heart.

TAPVC

Total anomalous pulmonary venous connection
Abnormal venous drainage of both lungs into right atrium. Four types: supracardiac, cardiac, infradiaphragmatic and mixed. Associated atrial septal defect (ASD) always present.
TAPVD, TAPVR
(see CHD, PAPVD)

TAPVD

Total anomalous pulmonary venous drainage
See under TAPVC.
TAPVR
(see CHD, PAPVD)

TAPVR

Total anomalous pulmonary venous return
See under TAPVC.
TAPVD
(see CHD, PAPVD)

TAR

Trans-anal resection
Surgical resection of low-lying rectal carcinoma via anal canal.

TAVB

Total atrio–venticular block
Failure of conduction of cardiac atrial electrical activity to the ventricles which requires pacing.
CHB

TB

Tracheobronchial
Relating to the principal airways.

TB, Tb

Tuberculosis
Chronic infection caused by *Mycobacterium tuberculosis*, characterized by granuloma formation and cell-mediated hypersensitivity. (*see AFB*)

TBB

Transbronchial biopsy
1. The procedure of sampling lung tissue through a bronchoscope.
2. The specimen obtained by this technique.

TBG

Thyroxine binding globulin
Plasma protein which binds thyroxine (T4).

TBI

Total body irradiation
Radiotherapy used to destroy diseased bone marrow prior to a bone marrow transplant.

$T_{\frac{1}{2}}$ biol

Biological half-life
Half-life for the reduction of activity of a radionuclide in the human body owing to biological processes, e.g. renal excretion. (*see $T_{\frac{1}{2}}$, $T_{\frac{1}{2}}phys$, $T_{\frac{1}{2}}eff$*)

TBLC

Term birth living child
Obstetric term for healthy child born after at least 38 weeks gestation.

TBPA

Thyroxine binding prealbumin
Protein binding thyroxine (T4) in the circulation.

TBV

Total blood volume
Total combined red cell and plasma volume.

TBW

Total body water
Total intra- and extracellular water in the body.

^{99m}Tc, 99m-Tc

Technetium-99m
Radionuclide commonly used for imaging in nuclear medicine. It may be bound to a tracer or used as its salt, pertechnetate (TcO_4^-).

T&C

Type and crossmatch
Determination of blood group and testing of donor red blood cells against recipient serum.
XM, X match

TC

Transverse colon
The segment of large bowel connecting the ascending and descending colon.

Tc

Correlation time
Describes random molecular motion.

TCA

Tricyclic antidepressants
Group of antidepressant drugs.

TCB

Transabdominal chorionic biopsy
Sampling of placental material using a percutaneous approach. Used in prenatal diagnosis of genetic disease.

TCC

Transitional cell carcinoma
Malignancy of the transitional cells which line the surface of urinary collecting system from renal pelvis to urethra.

TCCD

Transcranial colour coded Doppler
Imaging of blood flow within the infant head using Doppler ultrasound applied externally.
TCCS
(*see TCD*)

TCCS

Transcranial colour coded sonography
See under TCCD.
(*see TCD*)

TCD

Transcranial Doppler
Imaging of blood flow within the infant head, using Doppler ultrasound applied externally.
(*see TCCD*)

TCD

Transverse cardiac diameter
Sum of the maximum horizontal distances from an imaginary vertical line bisecting the heart to the right and left edges of the cardiac shadow on a standard six foot postero-anterior (PA) radiograph.

T cell

Thymus-derived cell
Lymphocyte of thymic origin, involved in the immune response.

TCG

Time compensated gain
Function on an ultrasound machine which amplifies echoes returning from deeper parts of body, so final ultrasound image is uniform at all depths.
TGC

TCI

To come in
Patient due for hospital admission.

TCLL

T cell lymphocytic leukaemia
Neoplastic proliferation of differentiated T lymphocytes which infiltrate bone marrow, spleen, lymph nodes and other organs, e.g. skin.

$^{99m}TcO_4^-$, TcO_4^-, $^{99m}TcO_4^-$

Technetium-99m pertechnetate
Salt of technetium-99m (^{99m}Tc) used unbound to any tracer for imaging various organs in nuclear medicine (e.g. thyroid).

TCP/IP

Transmission contrast protocol/Internet protocol
A transport and Internet working protocol which is a networking standard.

TCR

True count rate
Actual number of disintegrations per second, not those detected.

TD

Tabes dorsalis
Dorsal column demyelination in tertiary syphilis (3°Σ).

TD

Thoracic duct
Main lymphatic vessel in the body.

TDLU

Terminal ductal lobular unit
Anatomical term to describe the terminal branches in lobes of the breast, consists of extralobular terminal duct and lobule.

tds (US: ttd)

Ter die sumendum
To be taken three times a day.
tid

TE

Echo time
Time between the centre of an applied 90-degree pulse and the centre of the spin echo signal in magnetic resonance imaging.

TED

Thromboembolic disease
Abnormal formation and migration of blood clots within vessels.

TED stockings

Thromboembolic deterrent stockings
Tight support stockings preventing the development of deep vein thrombosis in patients at risk from this complication.

TEE (US)

Transesophageal echocardiography
Endoscopic ultrasound examination of the heart using an ultrasound probe in the oesophagus.
TOE

$T_{\frac{1}{2}}$eff

Effective half-life
Half-life for the overall reduction of activity of a radionuclide in the body owing to combined physical and biological processes.

TEM

Transmission electron microscope
Instrument for viewing objects too small to be resolved by light beams. Images are formed by electrons from a focused beam which passes through the specimen.
EM

Temp.

Temperature
Often synonymous with pyrexia.

TEN

Toxic epidermal necrolysis
Epidermal cell death in response to staphylococcal toxins or drug reaction. May be lethal.
STEN

TENS

Transcutaneous electrical nerve stimulation
Local pain relief using noninvasive electrical stimulation of skin surface.
TNS

TEP

Thromboembolism prophylaxis
Treatment to prevent intravascular clot formation.

Ter.

Tertiary
Third order.
3°

TEV

Talipes eqinovarus
Clubfoot. There is plantar flexion with inversion and adduction of the forefoot.

Texel

Texture element
The smallest part of an image texture (pattern) which, when it repeats in a certain way, makes up that texture.

TF

Tactile fremitus
Palpated voice vibrations communicated to the chest wall. Increased with consolidation, decreased with effusions.
TVF, VF
(see VR)

TFT

Thin film transistor
High quality type of display screen less subject to the flicker and drift seen with conventional cathode ray tube based screens.

TFTs

Thyroid function tests
Biochemical assessment of thyroid activity.

TG

Tocogram
Fetal heart rate monitor using Doppler ultrasound.
CTG

TGA

Transposition of the great arteries
Congenital cardiovascular anomaly with aorta arising from right ventricle and pulmonary artery arising from left ventricle.
TGV
(see CHD)

TGC

Time gain compensation
See under TCG.

TGV

Transposition of the great vessels
See under TGA.
(see CHD)

Th, T_h

T helper cell
Serum quantification of the circulating population of 'helper' T lymphocytes; intimately involved in immune defence. Low count in acquired immunodeficiency syndrome (AIDS).
CD4

THC

Tetrahydrocannabinoid
Cannabis derived anti-emetic.

Thor

Thorax, thoracic
Chest or chest wall.

THP

Trans-hepatic portography
Contrast examination of the hepatic portal vein performed by direct injection into liver.

tHPT

Tertiary hyperparathyroidism
Raised serum parathyroid hormone from an autonomously secreting adenoma. May develop in long-standing secondary hyperparathyroidism.
3° HPT

THR

Total hip replacement
Replacement of diseased hip joint with a prosthesis.

TI

Therapeutic index
Ratio of toxic dose or concentration of a drug to its therapeutic dose or concentration.

TI

Tricuspid incompetence / insufficiency
Cardiac valve disease, allowing retrograde flow across the tricuspid valve back into the right atrium during systole.
TR

TIA

Transient ischaemic attack
Sudden focal neurological deficit lasting less than 24 hours.
TRINS
(see PRIND, RIND)

Tib.

Tibia

Principal bone of the lower leg.

TIBC

Total iron binding capacity

Measure of the transferring (iron binding protein) level in plasma. Elevated in iron deficiency anaemia.

IBC

TICC

Time interval from cessation of contraception to conception

Assessment of fertility.

tid (US: ttd)

Ter in die

See under tds.

ttd

TIMI

Transmural inferior myocardial infarction

Full-thickness ischaemic death of cardiac tissue resulting from right coronary artery occlusion.

IMI

TIPJ

Terminal interphalangeal joint

Synomial joint between the middle and distal phalanges of hand or foot.

DIPJ

TIPS

Transjugular intrahepatic portosystemic shunt

Percutaneous placement of metallic stent between portal and hepatic veins within the liver for the treatment of portal hypertension.

TIPSS

TIPSS

Transjugular intrahepatic portosystemic stent shunt

See under TIPS.

TIS

Tumour *in situ*

Minute intraepithelial malignant foci often considered to constitute a precancerous state.

CIS

TJ

Triceps jerk

Involuntary contraction of triceps muscle in response to stretching of its tendon.

TKR

Total knee replacement

Replacement of a diseased knee with a prosthesis.

^{201}Tl

Thallium-201

Radionuclide used for visualization of myocardial perfusion.

201-Tl

TL

Thermoluminescence

Physical property of light emission in response to heating.

TL

Tubal ligation

Surgical tying of the Fallopian tube, usually for sterilization.

(*see Lap. Steri.*)

TLA

Translumbar aortography

Radiographic imaging of the aorta by means of the direct percutaneous injection of contrast medium into the lumbar aorta.

TLA

Transluminal angioplasty

See under TAP.

PTA

TLC

Tender loving care

Kind, supportive treatment.

TLC

Total lung capacity

Total volume of air in lungs following a maximal inspiration.

(*see FEV, IC, IRC, RV*)

TLC

Transverse loop colostomy

Surgically fashioned communication of the transverse colon with the exterior to bypass the distal colon.

TLD

Thermoluminescent dosimeter

Device for monitoring exposure (X) to staff working with ionizing radiation. Uses the principle of thermoluminescence.

TLL

T cell leukaemia / lymphoma

Malignant infiltration of blood, bone marrow and other tissues with abnormal T lymphocytes causing lymphadenopathy, hepatosplenomegaly and cutaneous infiltrations.

TLV

Total lung volume
See under TLC.

TM-MODE

Time-motion mode
Ultrasound technique recording variation of ultrasound amplitude and depth with time. Used in echocardiography.
M-MODE

TMA

Transmetatarsal amputation
Amputation of toes cutting through the metatarsal bones.

TMB

Transient monocular blindness
Brief episode of blindness due to temporary occlusion of the optic artery. Also known as *amaurosis fugax.*

TMI

Threatened myocardial infarction
Angina with rest pain.

TMJ

Temporomandibular joint
Synovial joint between skull and jaw.

TMR

Topical magnetic resonance
Spectroscopic technique that uses special shim coils to produce a small region of high field homogeneity.

TMTJ

Tarsometatarsal joint
Synovial joint between tarsal and metatarsal bones in the foot.

TN

Trigeminal neuralgia
Brief episodes of intense pain in the distribution of one or more branches of the trigeminal nerve (5th cranial nerve, CNV).

TN

True negative
Scientific observation correctly deemed to be negative in respect of a particular test. Used in patients with reference to diagnostic tests. Term used in statistics.
(see FN, FP, TP)

TNA

Total nail ablation
Operation to obliterate entire nailbed.

TNF

Tumour necrosis factor
Substance produced by macrophages with cytotoxic effects. A recombinant form is used to treat malignant melanoma.

TNI

Total nodal irradiation
Radiotherapy to all lymph nodes performed to achieve immune suppression prior to organ engraftment or to treat autoimmune diseases.

TNM

Tumour nodes metastases
Staging system used for all forms of malignancy indicating amount of local spread, presence of involved lymph nodes and distant metastases.

TNS

Transcutaneous nerve stimulation
See under TENS.

TO

Telephone order
Doctor's telephonic instruction, usually to give a drug.
(see Verbal)

TOE

Tender on examination
Pain elicited on physical examination of a part of the body.

TOE

Trans-oesophageal echography
See under TEE.

TOF

Tetralogy of Fallot
Complex congenital cardiovascular abnormality comprising ventricular septal defect, infundibular pulmonary arterial stenosis, right ventricular hypertrophy and over-riding aorta.
(see BT Shunt, CHD, FT)

TOF

Time of flight
Technique used for magnetic resonance angiography (MRA).

TOF

Tracheo–oesophageal fistula
Pathological connection between trachea and oesophagus, usually congenital.
(see OA, VACTER, VATER)

Tomo.

Tomogram
Imaging technique involving movement of imaging source and/or detector to provide enhanced diagnostic information in respect of the object plane in focus.

TOP

Termination of pregnancy
Surgical abortion.
STOP, TAB

TOPS

Take off pounds sensibly
Lose weight.

TORCH

Toxoplasmosis, other (commonly syphilis), rubella, cytamegalovirus and herpes simplex
Maternal infections acquired prenatally or perinatally, which may affect the fetus.

T&P

Temperature and pressure
Observations of body temperature and blood pressure.

T&P

Temperature and pulse
Observations of body temperature and pulse rate.

TP

Total protein
Measure of the total plasma protein. An elevated level is a non-specific marker for disease.

TP

True positive
Scientific observation correctly deemed to be positive in respect of a particular test. Used in patients with reference to diagnostic tests.
(*see FN, FP, TN*)

Tp

Primary transmission
Percentage of primary radiation transmitted through a grid. Tp = intensity (I) with grid / intensity without grid × 100.

TPA

Treponema pallidum **agglutination assay**
Test for active syphilis infection (Σ).
TPHA

tPA/TPA

Tissue plasminogen activator
Thrombolytic agent used in treatment of myocardial infarction and intravascular thrombosis.
(*see rtPA*)

TPAI

Tissue plasminogen activator inhibitor
Agent which counteracts the thrombolytic action of tissue plasminogen activator (tPA).

TPHA

Treponema pallidum **haemagglutination assay**
See under TPA.

$T_{\frac{1}{2}}$ phys

Physical half-life
Time after which the radioactivity of a substance has decayed to half its original value solely as a result of physical processes.
(*see $T_{\frac{1}{2}}$, $T_{\frac{1}{2}}biol$, $T_{\frac{1}{2}}eff$*)

TPI

Treponema pallidum **immobilization test**
Specific test for syphilis infection (Σ).

TPN

Total parenteral nutrition
Nutrition delivered solely by the intravenous route in cases where oral feeding is impossible or inadvisable.

TPR

Temperature, pulse, respiration
Routine observations of vital signs.
Obs

TPR

Total peripheral resistance
Opposition to blood flow offered by the entire systemic vascular tree.
PVR, SVR, TPVR, TSVR, TVR

TPVR

Total peripheral vascular resistance
See under TPR.
PVR, SVR, TSVR, TVR

TPVS

Transhepatic portal venous sampling
Percutaneous catheterization of the portal vein and selective catheterization of its tributaries to obtain blood samples for humoral assay. Principally used for the localization of small pancreatic endocrine tumours.

TQA, TQM

Total quality assessment / management
A structured systematic management
discipline which aims to improve quality and
efficiency.
(see CQI)

Trans.

Transverse section
Imaging in a plane at right angles to the
principal axis of a structure. Cross-sectional
imaging.
TLS, TS, Tsect, XS, X/S

t/r

Photoelectric mass attenuation coefficient
Coefficient for X or gamma ray (γ ray)
attenuation by photoelectric interaction per
unit mass. Depends on absorber material and
beam energy.
(see m/r, r)

TR

Time to repeat, repetition time, repeat time
Time between the beginning of one pulse
sequence and the next in magnetic resonance
imaging.

TR

Trans rectal
Via the anus and rectum.
PR

TR

Tricuspid regurgitation
See under TI.

TRACH

Trachea
Main airway extending from the larynx to the
carina.
(see CXR)

TRASHES

**Tuberculosis, radiotherapy, ankylosing
spondylitis, histoplasmosis, extrinsinc allergic
alveolitis, silicosis**
Radiological causes of upper zone fibrotic
changes on chest x-ray (CXR).
BREASTS

TRBF

Total renal blood flow
Volume of blood passing through the kidneys
in unit time.

T reflex

Tendon reflex
Involuntary contraction of a muscle in
response to stretching of its tendon.

TRH

Thyrotrophin-releasing hormone
Hormone produced by hypothalamus which
stimulates the anterior pituitary to produce
TSH.

TRINS

**Totally reversible ischaemic neurological
symptoms**
Sudden focal neurological deficit lasting less
than 24 hours.
TIA
(see PRIND, RIND)

tRNA

Transfer ribonucleic acid
Nucleic acid used in copying deoxyribonucleic
acid for cell replication.

TRO

To rule out
Exclude.
R/O

Troch.

Trochanter
Greater and lesser bony prominences on the
femur.

Truncus

Truncus arteriosus
See under TA.

TRUS

Trans rectal ultrasound
Ultrasonic imaging technique using a probe
inserted into the rectum.

TRVV

Total right ventricular volume
Volume of blood in the right ventricle at the
end of ventricular diastole.

TS

Takayasu's syndrome
Arteritis affecting aorta and other major
arteries which commonly causes stenosis or
occlusion. Also known as the aortic arch
syndrome or pulseless disease.

TS

Transsexual
1. Individual who identifies with the opposite
sex.
2. One who has undergone surgical gender
reassignation.

TS, T/S

Transverse section
See under Trans.
Tsect, XS, X/S

TS

Tricuspid stenosis
Narrowing of the tricuspid valve.

TSA

Tumour specific antigen
Antigen present only on tumour cells and
different from those expressed by normal cells.

TSD

Tay Sachs disease
Familial amaurotic idiocy. Autosomal
recessive gangliosidosis caused by deficiency
of lysosomal hexaminidase A. Causes
developmental delay, fits and death by
age 3–5.

Tsect

Transverse section
See under Trans.
TS, T/S, XS, X/S

TSG

Thyroid stimulating globulin
Hormone produced by the pituitary which
stimulates the thyroid to produce thyroxine.
TSH
(see TRH)

TSH

Thyroid stimulating hormone
See under TSG.
(see TRH)

tsp.

Teaspoon
Volume measure equivalent to 5 millilitres.

TSP

Tropical spastic paraperesis
Slowly progressive disease of the spinal cord
caused by infection with human T-cell
leukaemia virus 1 (HTLV-1). Occurs in
tropical regions of the Caribbean, South
America and Africa.

TSS

Toxic shock syndrome
Fever, rash, diarrhoea, severe myalgia and
shock caused by *Staphylococcus aureus* toxin,
occurs in a number of situations in all ages and
both sexes, but there is a particular association
with the use of Mg$^+$-chelating tampons in
menstruating women.

TSSD

Theatre sterile supply department
Centre for sterilization of operating theatre
equipment.
TSSU
(see CSSD, CSSU)

TSSU

Theatre sterile supply unit
See under TSSD.
(see CSSD, CSSU)

TSVR

Total systemic vascular resistance
See under TPR.
PVR, SVR, TPVR, TVR

TT

Tetanus toxoid
Antigenic material for active immunization
against tetanus.

TT

Thrombin time
One parameter used in the assessment of blood
coagulation status.

TTD

Thoracic transverse diameter
Widest horizontal distance between medial
aspects of ribs on a frontal chest radiograph
(CXR).

ttd

Three times daily
Directions for medication.
tds, tid

ttfo

Asked to leave hospital!
Refers to unpleasant patients.

TTP

Thrombotic thrombocytopenic purpura
Haematological disorder of unknown
aetiology, characterized by haemolytic
anaemia, thrombocytopenia, fever,
neurological disorders, and renal dysfunction.

TTS

Through the scope
Procedure performed through the biopsy
channel of an endoscope, e.g. placement of an
oesophageal dilatation balloon etc.

Tu.

Tumour
Neoplastic growth.
Neo., NG

T tube

'T'-shaped tube used for simultaneous internal and external biliary drainage.

turboFLASH

Turbo fast low angle shot

Ultrafast magnetic resonance imaging technique that employs a separate magnetization preparation period before a standard fast low angle shot (FLASH) sequence with a short repetition time.
MP-RAGE

TURB

Transurethral resection of the bladder

Surgical procedure to remove a bladder tumour, using a cystoscope.

TURBT

Transurethral resection of bladder tumour

See under TURB.

TURP

Transurethral resection of the prostate

Surgical procedure to remove prostatic tissue, using a urethroscope.

TUU

Transureteroureterostomy

End-to-side anastomosis of the proximal segment of a divided ureter to the contralateral ureter.

TV

Television

The system or process involved in the production of a series of transient images on a fluorescent screen using a cathode-ray tube.

TV

Tidal volume

The amount of gas exchanged during a single respiratory cycle.

TV

Trans vaginam

When applied to ultrasound, means a pelvic examination obtained by positioning an ultrasound probe in the vagina.
EVS, PV

TV

Transvestite

Person dressing in clothes of the opposite sex.

TV

Tricuspid valve

Heart valve between the right atrium and right ventricle.

TVCV

Transvenous cardioversion

Termination of a cardiac arrhythmia using an implantable device with electrodes passing through the superior vena cava to the right atrium and ventricle.

TVE

Tricuspid valve excursion

The movement of the tricuspid valve.

TVF

Tactile vocal fremitus

See under TF.
VF
(see VR)

TVL

Tenth value layer

Thickness of absorber required to reduce X or gamma ray intensity to one tenth of its original value.

TVMF

Time varying magnetic fields

Magnetic fields that change with time. They are necessary for image formation in MRI.

TVP

Truncal vagotomy and pyeloroplasty

Operation for peptic ulcer involving resection of part of both vagus nerves as they enter the abdomen combined with widening of the gastric outlet.
V&P

TVR

Total vascular resistance

See under TPR.
PVR, SVR, TPVR, TSVR

TVR

Tricuspid valve replacement / repair

Replacement or repair of diseased tricuspid valve.

TVRE

Transvaginal resection of endometrium

Surgical removal of endometrium through vagina.

TVS (US)

Transvesical sonography

Pelvic ultrasound performed transcutaneously via a probe on the lower abdominal wall, using the full bladder as a sonographic window.

TVU (US)

Total volume of urine
Volume of urine passed, usually over 24 hours.
UOP

T₁W, T1W

T₁ weighted
Denotes a magnetic resonance sequence,
demonstrating anatomy, timed to emphasize
the T_1 tissue characteristics in magnetic
resonance imaging (MRI).
(*see* T_1, T_1WI)

T₁W1, T1WI

T₁ weighted image
A magnetic resonance image (MRI), sensitive
to anatomy, produced using a sequence timed
to emphasize the T_1 tissue characteristics.
(*see* T_1, T_1W)

T₂W, T2W

T₂ weighted
Denotes a magnetic resonance sequence,
sensitive to pathology, timed to emphasize the
T2 tissue characteristics.
(*see* T_2, T_2WI)

TW

Travelling wave
Transfer of energy and momentum from a
source to surroundings.

TWA

Time weighted average
See under TAM.

T₂WI, T2WI

T₂ weighted image
A magnetic resonance image, sensitive to
pathology, produced using a sequence timed to
emphasize the T_2 tissue characteristics.
(*see* T_2, T_2W)

Tx

Treatment / therapy
Rx

Tx

Transplant
Organ transplanted from one individual into
another.

Tx

Transplantation
The removal of an organ from a donor and
insertion into a recipient.

Tx kidney

Transplant kidney
A kidney that has been transplanted from a
donor to a recipient.
KTx

Tymp.

Tympanic
Relating to the eardrum.

Typ.

Typical

Tyr.

Tyrosine
Amino acid produced from phenylalanine.

u/U
Units

U
Unsharpness / Total unsharpness
Degree of ill-definition of an edge on a radiograph. Geometric unsharpness (UG), movement unsharpness (UM), absorption unsharpness (UA), film/screen unsharpness (UF, US), and parallax unsharpness (UP) all contribute.
UT

U (US: BUN)
Urea
Excretion product of protein breakdown. The serum concentration of urea is an indicator of renal function.

UA
Absorption unsharpness
Blurring caused by a gradual change in X-ray absorption across the boundary or edge of an examined object.
(see U)

UA
Uric acid
End product of purine nucleotide metabolism in humans. An excess of uric acid is associated with gout.

UAC
Umbilical artery catheter
Catheter placed in the umbilical artery of neonates for measuring arterial pressure and blood gases.

UAP
Unstable angina pectoris
Cardiac ischaemic pain commonly occurring at rest or on minimal exertion, the pattern and/or nature of which shows deterioration from a previously more stable character. Associated with high risk of myocardial infarction.

UAPA
Unilateral absence of pulmonary artery
Absence of right or left main pulmonary artery.
(see CHD)

UBOs
Unidentified bright objects
High focal signals from subcortical cerebral white matter seen on magnetic resonance (MRI) brain images. Incidence increases with age. Diverse aetiology.
WMHs

UC
Ulcerative colitis
Chronic colonic inflammatory disorder of unknown aetiology.

UCD
Usual diseases of childhood
Common illnesses in children.
UCHD, UDC

UCG
Ultrasound cardiography
Imaging the heart using ultrasound.
Echo., USCG

UCG
Urinary chorionic gonadotrophin
Hormone produced by a fertilized ovum, can be used to confirm pregnancy.
(see βHCG)

UCHD
Usual diseases of childhood
See under UCD.
UDC

UCI
Urinary catheter in
Indwelling tube draining urine from the bladder.

Ucs
Unconscious
Unresponsive; insensible.

UD
Ulnar deviation
Angulation of digit(s) and or metacarpals towards the midline, with the arm in the anatomical position.

UD
Urethral dilatation
Procedure to relieve a urethral stricture.

UD
Urethral discharge
Abnormal excretion from the urethra.

UDC
Usual diseases of childhood
See under UCD.
UCHD

UDS

Ultrasound Doppler sonography
Evaluation of vascular flow using ultrasound.

U&E

Urea and electrolytes
Standard serum biochemistry test.

UE

Upper extremity
1. Arm
2. Upper limit of a lesion.

UES

Upper esophageal sphincter
Muscular junction between the pharynx and oesophagus

UF

Film unsharpness
Blurring caused by light diffusion in the film layer.
(*see U, US*)

UF

Ultrafiltration
Removal of water and solutes from blood in the glomeruli.

UF coll., UF collimator

Ultra fine collimator
High ratio collimator used for imaging detail.

UFC

Urinary free cortisol
Excretion product of cortisol, elevated in Cushing's syndrome.

UG

Geometric unsharpness
Caused by the penumbra of an object on a radiograph. The penumbra results from the finite size of the focal spot (F).
(*see U*)

UGI

Upper gastrointestinal
Pertaining to the oesophagus, stomach, duodenum and small intestine.

UGT

Urogenital tract
The excretory and genital organs.

UID

Unique image identifier
A specific 'label' which uniquely identifies a digital image in a computer database.

UIP

Usual interstitial pneumonitis
Progressive pulmonary fibrosis of an unknown cause.
CFA, FA, IPF
(*see DIP*)

UIQ

Upper inner quadrant
Supero-medial quarter, usually of the breast.

UKAEA

United Kingdom Atomic Energy Authority
Body regulating the production and use of radioactive substances.

UKAS

United Kingdom Association of Sonographers
British body of radiographers in ultrasound.

UL

Upper lobe
Superior division of either lung.

ULLE

Upper lid left eye

ULQ

Upper left quadrant
Non-anatomical term to describe left superior quarter of the abdomen (or breast).
LUQ

ULRE

Upper lid right eye

Ultrafast CT

Ultrafast computed tomography
Extremely fast computed tomography (CT) using a rapidly rotating electron beam and stationary circular anodes.
EBT

UM (US: MU)

Movement unsharpness
Caused by motion of the examined object (patient) during exposure. Patient unsharpness.
(*see U*)

UMN

Upper motor neurone / nerve
Central spinal motor nerve cell and processes.
(see LMN)

UMNL

Upper motor neurone lesion
Damage to the central spinal motor nerve.

UN

United Nations
International organization of independent states formed in 1945 to promote peace and international co-operation.

UNESCO

United Nations Educational, Scientific and Cultural Organization

UO

Ureteric orifice
Opening of the ureter into the bladder.

UO (US: TVU)

Urinary output
Volume of urine excreted during a specified period, usually 24 hours.
TVU, UOP

UOP

Urine output
See under UO.
TVU

UOQ

Upper outer quadrant
Supero-lateral quarter, usually of the breast.

U/P

Urine / plasma
Ratio of the concentrations of a substance in urine and plasma.

UP

Parallax unsharpness
Blurring caused by the separation of the two emulsions of a double emulsion film by the width of the film base.
(*see U*)

UPJ

Ureteropelvic junction
Anatomical boundary between the renal pelvis and proximal ureter.
PUJ

UQ

Upper quadrant
Descriptive division of body part.

Ur

Urea
See under U.

URL

Uniform resource locator
The specification of a network service or document. An address on the World Wide Web (WWW).

URQ

Upper right quadrant
Non-anatomical term to describe right superior quarter of the abdomen (or breast).
RUQ

URT

Upper respiratory tract
Pertaining to the airways above the pharynx.
(*see LRT*)

URTI

Upper respiratory tract infection
Infection of the upper airways, above the pharynx.
(*see LRTI*)

US

Screen unsharpness
Blurring due to light diffusion in the screen phosphor layer.
(*see U, UF*)

US

Ultrasound
Method of imaging using sound waves with a frequency above the normal audible range.
USS

USCG

Ultrasound cardiography
See under UCG.
Echo

USDEHW

United States Department of Health, Education and Welfare
American office for hospitals, schools and social services.

USS

Ultrasound scanning
See under US.

UT

Total unsharpness
See under U.
(*see UA, UF, UG, UM, UP, US*)

UT

Urinary tract
The kidneys, ureters, bladder and urethra.

UTI

Urinary tract infection
Infection of any part of the urinary tract.

UTO

Urinary tract obstruction
Obstruction to the flow of urine from either structural or functional causes.

UTP

Unshielded twisted pair
Insulated cable pairs without shielding. Their signals suffer noise degradation.

UUN

Urinary urea nitrogen
US term for concentration of urea in the urine.

UV

Ultraviolet
Electromagnetic radiation with a wavelength shorter than that in the visible range.
UVR
(see UVA, UVB, UVC)

UV

Umbilical vein
Vein in the umbilical cord, carrying oxygenated blood to the fetus, via the fetal left portal vein (PV), ductus venosus (DV) and inferior vena cava (IVC).

UVA

Ultraviolet A
Frequency band within the electromagnetic spectrum (320–380 nanometres).
(see UV)

UVB

Ultraviolet B
Frequency band within the electromagnetic spectrum (280–320 nanometres).
(see UV)

UVC

Ultraviolet C
Frequency band within the electromagnetic spectrum (10–280 nanometres).
(see UV)

UVC

Umbilical vein catheter
Catheter placed in the umbilical vein of neonates for circulatory support.

UVEB

Unifocal ventricular ectopic beat
Ventricular contraction without associated atrial electrical activity. Repeated beats all have the same appearance on an electrocardiogram.

UVJ

Ureterovesical junction
Anatomical division between the distal ureter and bladder.
VUJ
(see VUO)

UVR

Ultraviolet radiation
See under UV.

V1–6
Ventral 1 to 6
Anterior chest leads used in
electrocardiography.

v
Velocity
Rate of motion in a particular direction.

V
Fifth cranial nerve (trigeminal).
CV, CNV, CN5

V
Volt
SI unit of electrical potential.
(see eV, KeV, kV, kVp, MeV, MV)

V
Voltage
Electromotive force or potential difference
expressed in volts.

V&P
Vagotomy and pyeloroplasty
Operation for peptic ulcer involving resection
of part of both vagus nerves as they enter the
abdomen combined with widening of the
gastric outlet.
TVP

VACTER
**Vertebral, vascular, anorectal, cardiac,
tracheal, esophageal, renal/radial ray**
Association of congenital anomalies occurring
with tracheo-oesophageal fistula.
VACTERL, VATER
(see TOF)

VACTERL
**Vertebral/vascular, anorectal, cardiac,
tracheal, esophageal, renal/radial, limbs**
See under VACTER.
(see TOF)

VAS
**Ventricular atrial shunt / ventriculoatrial
shunt**
Connection between the cerebral ventricles
and the right atrium introduced to relieve
hydrocephalus.
(see VPS)

VATER
**Vertebral/vascular, anorectal, tracheal,
esophageal, renal/radial**
See under VACTER.
(see TOF)

VAW
Video acquisition workstation
Unit which converts images produced as a
video signal (e.g. ultrasound) into digital
format, displays them and sends them to a
picture archiving and communication system
(PACS).

VBI
Vertebrobasilar insufficiency
Hypoperfusion of that part of the brain
supplied by the vertebro-basilar arterial system.

VC
Vital capacity
Maximum volume of gas which can be expired
from lung following a maximal inspiration.

VCR
Vincristine
A dimeric alkaloid chemotherapeutic drug
used to treat leukaemia and lymphomas.

VD
Venereal disease
Sexually acquired infection.
STD

VD
Ventouse delivery
Delivery of a baby with the help of a Ventouse
suction device.

VDRL
Venereal disease research laboratory (test)
Serological screening test for syphilis (Σ).

VDT
Video display terminal
Basic dumb terminal (screen and keyboard)
used for user access to computer system.

VDU
Video display unit
Screen for viewing computer output.

VE
Ventricular ectopic / extrasystole
Premature cardiac beat originating in the
ventricles rather than the sinu-atrial node.
VPB

VEP

Visual evoked potential
Study of electrical activity in the brain in response to specific visual stimuli recorded by electrodes placed over the posterior portion of the scalp. Often abnormal in optic neuritis, raising the suspicion of multiple sclerosis.
PSVER, VER

VER

Visual evoked responses
See under VEP.
PSVER

Verbal

Verbal order
Doctor's instruction (spoken directly or over the telephone), usually to give a drug.
(see TO)

VG

Very good

VF

Ventricular fibrillation
Disordered fast cardiac electrical conduction, leading to cardiac arrest.

VF

Vocal fremitus
Palpated voice vibrations communicated to the chest wall. Increased with consolidation, decreased with effusions.
TF, TVF
(see VR)

VGA

Video graphics display
The entry-level standard for graphics display.

v.i.

vide infra
Latin for: 'see below'. Textual annotation.

VI

Sixth cranial nerve (abducens).
CNVI, CN6

VII

Seventh cranial nerve (facial).
CNVII, CN7

VIII

Eighth cranial nerve (vestibulocochlear).
CNVIII, CN8

VIN

Vulval intra-epithelial neoplasia
Non-invasive abnormal changes in cells of the vulva regarded as precursors of malignancy.

VIP

Vasoactive intestinal polypeptide
A hormone secreted by VIPoma tumours causing the syndrome of watery diarrhoea, hypokalaemia and dehydration.

VIPoma

Vasoactive intestinal peptide-secreting tumour
Pancreatic islet-cell tumour producing vasoactive intestinal peptide (VIP), a hormone causing the syndrome of watery diarrhoea, hypokalaemia, and dehydration.

virol.

Virology
Study of viral diseases and viruses.

viz.

videlicet
Latin: Textual annotation meaning 'namely' or 'as shown in this format'.

VLB

Vinblastin
A dimeric alkaloid chemotherapeutic drug used to treat leukaemia and lymphomas.

VLDL

Very low density lipoprotein
High molecular weight particle transporting triglycerides from liver to the cells.
(see IDL, LDL)

VMA

Vanillyl mandelic acid
Adrenaline metabolite. When present in urine is indicative of phaeochromocytoma.
(see HMMA)

VOD

Veno-occlusive disease
Cause of hepatic venous outflow obstruction involving the central and sublobular hepatic veins within the liver.

Voxel

Volume element
The smallest part of a three dimensional image volume.

VP

Variegate porphyria

Defect of porphyrin metabolism characterized by acute attacks of neuropsychiatric dysfunction and skin sensitivity to light.

VPB

Ventricular premature beat

See under VE.

VPC

Ventricular premature complex

Early cardiac electrical impulse initiating ventricular ectopic beat.

VPS

Ventricular peritoneal shunt

Connection between cerebral ventricles and peritoneal cavity introduced to relieve hydrocephalus.
(see VAS)

V/Q scan (US: V-P scan)

Ventilation perfusion scan

Pulmonary imaging technique for the evaluation of ventilation and perfusion by means of the intravenous injection of radioactive particles and the inhalation of radioactive gas. Often used to diagnose pulmonary embolism (PE).
(see ^{81m}-Kr, MAA)

VR

Virtual reality

Computer simulation of three dimensional space.

VR

Vocal resonance

Auscultated voice vibrations communicated to the chest wall. Increased with consolidation, decreased with effusions.
(see TF, TVF, VF)

VRE

Vancomycin resistant *enterococcus*

Mutant form of bacterium *enterococcus* resistant to many antibiotics including vancomycin.

VRS

Virchow–Robin Spaces

Perivascular subarachnoid spaces surrounding penetrating arteries as they enter basal ganglia or cortical grey matter.

VRT

Volume rendering technique

A reconstruction algorithm used to generate three dimensional (3D) computed tomography (CT) images.
(see MIP, SSD)

v.s.

vide supra

Latin for 'see above'.

VSD

Ventricular septal defect

Deficiency of wall between right and left ventricles.
(see ASD, CHD)

VSE

Volume-selective excitation

Spectroscopic technique that uses frequency-selective radiofrequency pulses to provide localization of spectra.

VT

Ventricular tachycardia

Cardiac arrhythmia defined as a run of at least three ventricular extrasystoles at a rate in excess of 120 beats per minute.

Vt

Tidal volume

Volume of air exchanged during single respiratory cycle.

VTEC

Verotoxin-producing *Escherichia coli*

Strains of *Escherichia coli* (*E.coli*) producing a toxin which is cytotoxic to monolayer cultures of Vero cells. May cause haemolytic uraemic syndrome (HUS) in children.
(see EIEC, EHEC, EPEC, ETEC)

VTOP

Vaginal termination of pregnancy

Induced abortion of fetus through the vagina.

VUJ

Vesico–ureteric junction

Anatomical division between distal ureter and bladder.
UVJ

VUO

Vesico–ureteric orifice

Opening of ureter into urinary bladder.
(see UVS, VUJ)

VV

Varicose veins

Dilated, tortuous superficial veins.

VWD

Von Willebrand's disease

Haematological bleeding disorder due to low
factor VIII clotting activity. Autosomal
dominant inheritance.

VZ

Varicella zoster

Herpes virus causing chicken pox and shingles.
Severe infection occurs in the immuno-
compromised.
HZ, HZV, VZV

VZV

Varicella zoster virus

See under VZ.
HZ, HZV

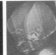

W

w, Ω
Ohm
SI unit of resistance (R).

W (US: Wolfram (G))
Tungsten (Wolfram)
Main constituent metal of most X-ray tube
anodes.
(see Rh)

W
Watt
SI unit of power. 1 W = 1 joule (J)/second (s)
$(1J\ s^{-1})$.
(see J, kW, s)

W
Week
Seven days.
wk, Wk, 6/52

WABU
Wash and brush up
Review/thorough check-up of patient with
known chronic disease, usually as a hospital
admission.

WAIS
**Western Angiographic and Interventional
Society (USA)**
US society for those specializing in
angiography and interventional radiology.
(see APSCVIR, BSIR, CIRSE, JSAIR, SCVIR)

WAN
Wide area network
Computer systems and terminals on distant
geographical sites, interconnected by
telephone links.

WAS
Wiskott–Aldridge syndrome
X-linked, recessively inherited
immunodeficiency disorder with eczema,
infections and thrombocytopenic
haemorrhage.

WASP (US)
White anglo-saxon protestant
North American descriptive term.

WB
Weight bear(ing)
Capable of bearing body weight. Refers to limb
or splint (e.g. plaster of Paris, POP).

WBC
White blood cell
Leucocyte (granulocyte, lymphocyte or
monocyte).

WBC
White blood count
Quantitation of white cell population in
serum.
WC, WCC

WC
Window centre
Centering point for grey scale when viewing
digitally produced images.
WL
(see WW)

WC
White count
Quantitation of white cell population in
serum, urine, cerebrospinal fluid (CSF) or
other body fluid.
(see WBC)

WCC
White cell count
See under WC.
(see WBC)

WCD
Weber–Christian disease
Non suppurative nodular panniculitis causing
skin nodules and multi-system involvement.
HWCD

WD
Withdrawn
Usually in relation to a drug no longer in use.

WDHA
**Watery diarrhoea, hypokalaemia and
achlorhydria**
Symptoms of Verner-Morrison syndrome,
which is caused by hypersecretion of
vasoactive intestinal peptide (VIP).
WDHH

WDHH
**Watery diarrhoea, hypokalaemia and
hypochlorhydria**
See under WDHA.

WE

Wernicke's encephalopathy
Nutritional thiamine deficiency, often in chronic alcoholics, characterized by ophthalmoplegia, ataxia and confusion.

WES

Wall echo sign
Characteristic appearance of a gall bladder full of stones, with a line of echoes from the gall bladder wall and a second line from stones packed tightly within the gall bladder.

WF

White female
Caucasian woman.

WFR

Weil–Felix reaction
Traditional serological test for typhus fever based on heterophil antibodies.

WFS

Waterhouse–Friedrichsen's syndrome
Adrenal cortical haemorrhage associated with meningococcal septicaemia.

WG

Wegener's granulomatosis
Generalized necrotizing vasculitis of medium-sized vessels predominantly affecting the upper respiratory tract, lungs and kidneys.

WHO

World Health Organization
International body setting standards and sponsoring improvements in health care.

WHR

Waist:hip ratio
Numerical comparison of waist and hip dimensions, indicator of fat distribution. Potential indicator for susceptibility to ischaemic heart disease.

wk, Wk

Week
Seven days.
w, 6/52

WKD

Wilson–Kimmelsteil disease
Diffuse or nodular renal glomerulosclerosis in diabetic nephropathy.
KWD, KWS
(see GN)

WL, W/L

Waiting list
Patients not yet given appointments for attendance at, or admission to, hospital.

WL

Window level
See under WC.
(see WW)

WLE

Wide local excision
Surgical removal of a lesion and a substantial rim of normal tissue surrounding it.

WM

White male
Caucasian man.
Cauc.

WM

White matter
Macroscopic description of the myelinated elements in the central nervous system (CNS).
(see GM)

WMH

White matter hyperintensities
High focal signals from subcortical cerebral white matter seen on magnetic resonance (MR) brain images. Increased incidence with age. Diverse aetiology.
UBOs

WNL

Within normal limits
Descriptive of diagnostic tests or physical examination.
NAD

w/o

Without

WORM

Write once read many
Digital information which can be written only once onto a storage medium, but accessed many times.

WP

Word processor / processing
Software package designed for the creation and editing of text-based documents.

WPW

Wolff–Parkinson–White syndrome
Re-entry tachycardia caused by anomalous atrioventricular myocardial connection (Bundle of Kent).

WR

Wassermann reaction
Serological test for syphilis (Σ) indicative of active disease.

WR

Widal reaction
Serological test for typhoid and paratyphoid.

wrt

with respect to
Concerning.

ws, WS

Water soluble
Dissolves in water.

WSC

Water soluble contrast
A radiological contrast medium (CM) which is dissolvable in water.

WSU

Working storage unit
Device for short term digital image storage.
Type of redundant array of inexpensive discs (RAID).

WT

(Tissue) weighting factor
The proportion of the total cancer risk assigned to a particular organ when the whole body is uniformly irradiated. It expresses different radiation sensitivities of individual tissues and is used to calculate the effective dose equivalent (EDE).
(see QF, Sv)

w/v

Weight for volume
Proportions of a pharmaceutical solution or suspension.

w/w

Weight for weight
Proportions of a pharmaceutical preparation.

WW

Window width
Range of shades of grey selected for viewing a particular digital image.

WWW

World Wide Web
An ethernet computer network connecting computers around the world, allowing their users to share information with each other.

WYSIWYG

What you see is what you get
The (computer) screen displays documents exactly as they will appear when printed out.

 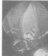

x′

Dimension in stationary frame of reference in magnetic resonance orthogonal to both the direction of static magnetic field z and to the y plane.

x

Dimension in the rotating frame of reference in plane orthogonal to both the direction of the static magnetic field (z) and to the y plane.

X

Radiation exposure
Total charge of ions of one sign produced by photons in air when all liberated electrons have been completely stopped. Unit: 1 Coulomb (C) / kilogram (kg) (Ckg^{-1}).

X

Tenth cranial nerve (vagus)
CNX, CX

x

Unknown quantity

^{127}Xe, 127-Xe

Xenon-127
Radioactive gas sometimes used for assessing ventilation in ventilation perfusion (V/Q) scans. Expensive and not widely available.
(see ^{133}Xe)

^{133}Xe, 133-Xe

Xenon-133
Radioactive gas used for assessing ventilation in ventilation perfusion (V/Q) scans. Also used to demonstrate bullae and air trapping.

Xe

Xenon
1. Gas used in ionization chambers for computed tomography (CT) and ionography chambers.
2. Radionuclides used for pulmonary imaging and vascular shunt measurement.
(see ^{127}Xe and ^{133}Xe)

XGP

Xanthogranulomatous pyelonephritis
Chronic suppurative granulomatous infection in chronic urinary obstruction originating in the medulla of the kidney.

XI

Eleventh cranial nerve (accessory)
CXI, CNXI

XII

Twelfth cranial nerve (hypoglossal)
CXII, CNXII

XM

Crossmatch
Determination of blood group and testing of donor red blood cells against recipient serum.
T&C, X match

Xmas factor

Christmas factor
Coagulation factor IX, deficiency of which causes haemophilia B.

X match (US: T&C)

Crossmatch
See under XM.
T&C

XO

Turner's syndrome
Syndrome characterized by primary amenorrhoea, sexual infantilism, short stature, multiple congenital anomalies and bilateral streak gonads in women lacking an X chromosome.

XP

Xeroderma pigmentosa
Autosomal recessive photosensitive skin disorder with macules, telangiectasia, keratoses and increased risk of cutaneous malignancy.

X Prep

X Prep
Commercial name of a laxative mixture used to prepare the bowel for contrast examinations.

XR

Xeroradiography
Edge-enhanced radiographic imaging using a charged selenium plate on which a latent image is formed by exposure to transmitted ionizing radiation.

X-ray

X-ray
1. Form of electromagnetic radiation.
2. Radiograph.
3. Radiographic procedure.
4. Department of radiology.
(see EM radiation; γray)

XS, X/S

Cross section
Imaging in a plane normal to the long axis of a structure; transverse section.
Trans., TS, T/S, Tsect

XS

Excess
Too much.

XU

Excretion urography
Basic radiographic method for examination of the urinary tract, using an intravenous injection of contrast medium.
IVP, IVU

XX

Female karyotype
Represents the two X chromosomes of the female.

XXY

Klinefelter's syndrome
Syndrome characterized by small, firm testes, azoospermia, gynaecomastia and elevated plasma gonadotrophin in men with two or more X chromosomes.

XY

Male karyotype
Represents the X and Y chromosomal pattern of the male.

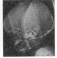

z

Dimension in the direction of static magnetic field in both the static and rotating frame of reference.

Z

Acoustic impedance of a material which determines its characteristics with respect to ultrasound beams.

Z

Atomic number
Number of protons matched by an equal number of electrons defining a specific element.
(*see A*)

ZDV

Zidovudine
Drug which inhibits the human immunodeficiency virus (HIV) in both symptomatic and asymptomatic patients.
AZT
(*see AIDS*)

ZEPI

Zonal echo planar imaging
Rapid acquisition magnetic resonance sequence used to demonstrate flowing blood.

ZES

Zollinger–Ellison syndrome
Disorder characterized by hypersecretion of gastrin.

Z Line

Zig-zag line
Border between the squamous and columnar epithelium at the oesophagogastric junction (OGJ).

ZN

Ziehl–Neelsen
Stain used for the microbiological demonstration of acid-fast bacilli (AFB), the cause of tuberculosis (TB).

(ZnCd)S

Zinc-cadmium sulphide
Phosphor commonly used for output fluorescent screens of image intensifiers (II). Also found as input fluorescent screens in older II.
(*see CsI*)

Symbols

\#

Fracture

Symbol commonly used to denote a fracture in conjunction with bone(s) involved.

<

Less than

≤

Less than or equal to

>

Greater than

≥

Greater than or equal to

↑

Raised level of/increased

↓

Decreased level of/decreased

[ ]

Denotes concentration/level of

~

Approximately

≈

Approximately

≅

Approximately

≡

Equivalent to

†

Death

Request forms

♂

male

♀

female

⊙

Unit or pint (of blood, saline, plasma etc.)

6/24

Hours (e.g. 6)

Duration in hours.

6/7

Days (e.g. 6)

Duration in days.

6/52

Weeks (e.g. 6)

Duration in weeks.

6/40

Weeks (e.g. 6) pregnant

Dating of standard 40 week human pregnancy.

6/12

Months (e.g. 6)

Duration in months.

α, **A**

Alpha

Proportional to.

β, **B**

Beta

γ, Γ

Gamma

δ, Δ

Delta

Diagnosis (medical). Difference or change (scientific).

ε, E

Epsilon

ζ, Z

Zeta

η, H

Eta

θ, Θ

Theta

ι, I

Iota

κ, K

Kappa

λ, Λ

Lambda

μ, M

Mu

ν, N

Nu

ξ, Ξ

Xi

o, O

Omicron

π, Π

Pi

↑Πθ

Hyperparathyroidism

↓Πθ

Hypoparathyroidism

ρ, P

Rho

σ, Σ

Sigma
Used as an abbreviation for syphilis and for
sigmoid colon.

τ, T

Tau

υ, Y

Upsilon

φ, Φ

Phi

χ, X

Chi

ψ, Ψ

Psi

ω, Ω

Omega
Symbol for resistance in ohm (Ω). Symbol for
Larmor frequency (W_o) of precession in
magnetic resonance.

c̄

with
See under *cum*.

@

at

°

degree

1°

primary

2°

secondary

3°

tertiary

−ve

negative

+ve

positive

R_x

Treatment or therapy
Abbreviation for Latin 'recipe', meaning
receive or take (as in a prescriptive).
(see Rx)